SLEEP WISE

SLEEP WISE

HOW TO FEEL BETTER, WORK SMARTER, AND BUILD RESILIENCE

DANIEL JIN BLUM, PHD
WITH EMILY TSIANG

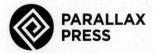
PARALLAX PRESS

BERKELEY, CALIFORNIA

Parallax Press
P.O. Box 7355
Berkeley, California
94707
parallax.org

Parallax Press is the publishing division of Unified Buddhist Church, Inc.

Disclaimer: This book is not intended as a substitute for the medical advice of physicians.
The reader should regularly consult a physician in matters relating to his/her health and
particularly with respect to any symptoms that may require diagnosis or medical attention.

Cover and text design by Josh Michels
Illustrations and patterns © Josh Michels
Author photos © Andrew Satanapong

Printed on 100% post-consumer waste recycled paper

Library of Congress Cataloging-in-Publication Data is available upon request

ISBN 978-1-941529-40-9

1 2 3 4 5 / 20 19 18 17 16

May this book put you to sleep

CONTENTS

MY SLEEP JOURNEY

"I now see how owning our story and loving ourselves through that process is the bravest thing that we will ever do."

—Brené Brown[1]

We all have a sleep story, a narrative about our own relationship to sleep. Our minds naturally weave facts and emotions from our past into narratives that help us remember and make sense of our experiences, contribute to our sense of self, and ultimately motivate us into action.

Since this is a book on sleep, I want to start with the sleep story we tell ourselves—a narrative about our own relationship to sleep. If we take time to reflect on our sleep story, what sleep actually *means* to us, we can then, with an open mind, take a look at which parts of our sleep story still serve us and which may not. When confronted with life's challenges, it is easy to become focused on finding a quick fix—drastic diets, crazy new exercise routines, or the "Five Simple Steps for a Good Night's Sleep"—and to overindulge in information-gathering and underinvest in reflection. When we build simple awareness of ourselves and our experiences, we can instead observe our stories as they unfold, allowing us the choice to follow the old pathways or to choose new ones. This is the first step in repairing and becoming wise about our sleep.

If, during this process, you find that you are satisfied with your sleep, cultivating awareness around it can heighten your enjoyment of it. If your sleep is not what you'd like it to be, examining how your stories contribute to your sleep can help you to select more supportive practices. The goal is not necessarily to change your sleep patterns, but rather to examine your own sleep story and how it influences the entirety of your life.

ONE OF THE LUCKY ONES

My own story begins with being told by my parents that I was a "good" sleeper, informed by my natural ability to get a high *quantity* of sleep. As a child, I could fall asleep the moment my head hit the pillow, and I usually slept as many hours as my schedule would allow. I could fall asleep anywhere—in the car, on the plane, even at school.

One of my family's favorite tales highlights my ability to sleep through anything. I grew up in Colorado, a Korean adoptee of parents who were avid outdoor enthusiasts. Each summer, they would take my brother, my two sisters, and me backpacking in the Rocky Mountains; we'd spend the day hiking into a remote site in the high mountains and then immerse ourselves in the endless wilderness. It was on one of these trips, after we had all retreated to our tents for the night, that a black bear came through our campsite. As you can imagine, it terrified my siblings and my parents. I, on the other hand, snored, reliably, through the whole episode. It didn't matter how many times they tried waking me up—my need for sleep overrode my fear of being eaten.

So it's no surprise that the running narrative I had for most of my life was: *I sleep so well that I can sleep through an earthquake; I must be one of the lucky ones.*

MY INTRODUCTION TO SLEEP MEDICINE

As I got older, my positive relationship with sleep nurtured my fascination with it. What happens when we sleep? How much sleep do we need? Why do we dream? While these were personally interesting quandaries, it never crossed my mind, even in the early years of my training as a psychologist, that there might be an entire specialty called sleep medicine that explored sleep health—in my professional field, no less.

Luckily, I was exposed to sleep as a treatment approach early on in my career. I had just arrived at Kearny Mesa Juvenile Hall, San Diego's main detention center for incarcerated youth, inspired to apply my burgeoning psychotherapy knowledge to help young people manage depression, anxiety, and trauma. My supervisor, Dr. Ilona Vail, asked me to shadow her on one of the sleep groups she facilitated in the highest-security unit; known as the 800 unit, it housed the most serious offenders. When she first mentioned these sessions, I looked at her and nodded thoughtfully like the good intern I was. But privately, I thought to myself: *Sleep groups? Does she mean we'll be watching them sleep? How awkward.*

As we walked down the hallway, she gave a quick rundown of the sessions: sleep hygiene (habits conducive to sleeping well) followed by deep breathing, progressive muscle relaxation, and guided visualization. I thought, *Sounds calming, but I'm not sure how this is going to help the guys on the 800 unit. They're looking at up to life in prison. Besides, these are teenagers. They're too self-conscious to try mindfulness exercises lying next to each other.* Fortunately, I kept all these thoughts to myself, because what I saw that day amazed me and blew away all my preconceptions. Not only did they fall asleep during the sessions, but the occurrence of violent outbreaks in the unit significantly decreased. It was such an obvious shift in behavior that the probation officers requested that we facilitate these sleep groups in other units as well.

Up to this point, I had been trained in psychotherapy, more commonly known as talk therapy. Often stereotyped by an image of a client lying on a therapist's couch, therapy can take numerous forms to help one process painful emotions, enhance interpersonal relationships, or change damaging patterns of behavior. Developing healthy behavior habits takes time and effort. It's a gradual process that requires moving through a series of conscious and unconscious stages of change—changes that our brains are hardwired to resist. To both the client and therapist, progress doesn't always feel tangible in the moment.

With the juvenile sleep groups, it was so clear. We witnessed an immediate reduction in their stress levels as they slowed their breath, disengaging them from the emotional centers of their brains and, ultimately, reducing their emotional manifestations of anxiety and anger. All of this was contained in a very safe space; an innocuous session of relaxation therapy introduced as *sleep,* a word free from the social stigmas associated with traditional therapy. This transformative experience would plant the seed in my thinking that treating sleep was not only an integral aspect of emotional well-being but also an underlying factor of overall health.

An Integrative Approach

As a psychologist, my approach had focused on addressing my clients' issues through empathy and insight, but these discoveries about the power of sleep and mindfulness led me to take a step back to explore the question: *How do our daily activities affect our minds and our moods?*

I knew that more exercise was better for your health, but I did not know that regular exercise could improve clinical depression. I knew that drinking plenty of water was good for you, but not that it could improve your mood and sleep. I intuitively knew that what we do to our bodies has profound effects on our minds, but it was not a connection that I had seriously considered exploring with my clients. I was used to a disorder-focused model of health care: the approach focused on treating the symptoms rather than the complete person and the dynamic interaction between their physical, psychological, social, and cultural dimensions.

As a clinician, the seemingly basic knowledge that we should adopt an integrated approach struck me hard because of how often I would sit with students who were struggling with depression or anxiety but were not taking care of the basics of sleep, nutrition, and exercise. Under Dr. Paula Andrasi's guidance at Western Michigan University's Counseling Center, I began to establish my core conceptualization of sleep and well-being as interrelated. The college students I saw usually had the ability to satisfy these needs in a basic way but lacked the knowledge of the benefits that establishing *good* sleep, nutrition, and exercise would bring. The more I helped these students explore sleep as part of their mental and global health, the more I shifted toward a holistic perspective, aiming to calm the mind through greater balance of the body.

All Snoring Is Abnormal

While my practice became more integrative, it lacked the comparable depth of therapeutic skills. I sought to deepen my professional understanding of sleep and enrolled in Stanford University's School of Sleep Medicine. This simple act would soon change the course of my own life.

On the first day of class, I learned that *all* snoring is abnormal and may be a sign of sleep apnea, a chronic condition in which a person stops breathing for brief periods while asleep. This disruption in sleep patterns can move one out of deep sleep and into light sleep, leading to poor sleep quality and excessive daytime sleepiness. What an insight! For my entire life, I had been told by family, friends, and popular culture that snoring was a sign of normal deep sleep. Snoring was part of my identity as a "good" sleeper. As the sleep-medicine class delved deeper, I learned that difficulties with recalling information, feeling overwhelmingly sleepy during the day, and falling asleep during classes were not just normal, occasional bouts of sleepiness—they were signs of chronic sleep deprivation. And they were all symptoms that both my partner, Emily, and I experienced on a daily basis.

This was revelatory stuff. My story began to unravel. I began to realize that my sleep, regardless of how much I got, was suboptimal. That it was not only the quantity of sleep that mattered, but also the quality of sleep. That I was actually one of the *un*lucky ones. The gears in my head began to click. *Was my snoring a sign that I had a sleep disorder?*

Getting Diagnosed

What began as a professional interest had suddenly become very personal. I immediately signed up for a sleep test and, sure enough, I was diagnosed with mild sleep apnea. The physician handed me a tennis ball and 2" PVC pipe, and said, "Sleep on your side and you'll be fine." *Wait, that's all? You've got to be kidding me.*

I had expected some sophisticated treatment and instead I was told to sleep with a tennis ball stuck to my back so I'd be forced to side-sleep. Not only did it feel ridiculous, but after trying it for several weeks, I continued to feel unrested. The positional treatment, to say the least, was uninspiring and disappointing. So I stopped. *It's mild sleep apnea, I'll be fine. A little sleepiness never hurt anyone. I can sleep in on the weekends.*

This rationalization completely discounted not only the potential long-term health consequences of my sleep disorder, such as heart disease and diabetes, but also the potential danger to myself and others if left untreated. For just one example, a recent study showed that clients with sleep apnea were 2.5 times more likely to be the driver in a car accident. But the discomfort of the tennis ball far outweighed the increased health risks, and it all seemed so intangible. I was 28 at the time of my diagnosis and still felt like I could function at a high level—completing a doctoral program, playing soccer several times a week, and testing normal on my physicals. I knew intellectually and professionally that any intervention would be challenging in the beginning, yet I was still resisting it. Even though I was a sleep psychologist, I was no exception; finding the motivation to change felt out of reach.

This dance with denial continued comfortably for a few months. I was finishing my post-doc in Michigan while Emily was in California. There was no one to hear me snore at night, and, therefore, no one to pester me about my sleep issues. That abruptly changed when I moved to San Francisco and moved in with her.

Instead of peacefully sleeping through the night, I'd wake up to find Emily fiercely pumping on my chest, saying, "You're not breathing!" It was as if I was having a cardiac arrest and she was performing nocturnal CPR. *It's just something strange that happens, but I feel fine so I must be okay.* Here

I was, being told that I regularly stopped breathing, and I continued to rationalize it as unrelated to my sleep apnea. The story I told myself—that I was a good sleeper, that snoring meant deep sleep—was so strong that I had convinced myself otherwise. Sleep had been so easy and enjoyable for me that I did not think it was something I needed to fix. It was hard to move past my initial sleep story.

My Partner in Sleep Apnea

For many of my clients, it's their partners who identify that something is wrong with their sleep. And it's their partners who provide the strength to come in for the treatment process: getting them in, supporting them, and helping hold them accountable. It was the same for me.

Emily, who actually did sleep through a 6.7 earthquake, was going through her own sleep evaluation at Stanford's Center for Sleep. Her sleep apnea diagnosis validated and explained all of the symptoms that had plagued her for years: frequent morning headaches, difficulty recalling information, and intense autoimmune episodes, such as eczema, allergies, and arthritis. She tried a CPAP (continuous positive airway pressure) machine and eventually opted for the more invasive treatment of maxillomandibular (jaw) advancement surgery and orthodontia. Within weeks of her surgery, she felt like she had a renewed lease on life.

As I watched Emily undergo these treatments and experience dramatic improvements, it became harder to ignore how crucial it was to address my own sleep issues. The continued sleepiness, my growing professional interest in sleep medicine, and my desire to spend more time with my partner awake and alert instead of asleep and drowsy inspired me to renew my efforts at improving my sleep. I began treatment with CPAP but, like Emily, eventually chose to pursue the maxillomandibular surgery myself. Most people with sleep apnea don't choose to undergo surgery; it is not a first-line treatment for several reasons. While it can provide comparable results to the CPAP, the surgery is quite painful, and it may not fully resolve the negative impact of your sleep apnea. After carefully weighing the pros and cons, I ultimately decided to opt for surgery because it offered the best opportunity to improve the quality of my relationship with sleep.

After the surgery, I felt amazing. My sleep was better than at any other point in my life. Even during the five weeks of recovery, I could feel a huge difference: my energy and exuberance remained about the same, but I no longer felt fatigued or sleepy during the day. I no longer needed nine to ten hours of sleep every night, nor did I feel sleepy for several hours after awakening. For the first time in my life, I could begin to reliably get up and go to the gym before work, something that had been absolutely unthinkable beforehand.

FULL CIRCLE

As the quality of my sleep continued to improve, my journey into sleep medicine expanded. I became a sleep coach at UC Berkeley's Sleep and Mood Research Clinic. Under the guidance of Dr. Allison Harvey, a preeminent sleep psychologist who leads the clinic and has been instrumental in shaping my trajectory in sleep medicine, I began providing cognitive behavioral therapy for insomnia (CBTi) in one of her longitudinal National Institute of Health–funded studies. I was excited to begin implementing these wonderfully effective tools and employing them with the intention of addressing the sleep, mood, and performance of teens.

Additionally, I returned to Stanford's Center for Sleep as a behavioral sleep medicine fellow, where I had the privilege to work alongside the fathers of sleep medicine, Dr. William Dement and Dr. Christian Guilleminault. It was at Stanford, the first sleep center in the world, that I went from student to client to clinical fellow. It really has felt like my sleep story, and my evolution as a sleep psychologist, has come full circle.

THIS BOOK

This book's title, *Sleep Wise,* reflects my perspective that each of us has the agency and the inner awareness to unlock our own story; it is within our own experiences that we can best shepherd ourselves toward a fuller, healthier life.

Guided by my learnings at both UC Berkeley and Stanford, this book illuminates the science and research behind sleep, nutrition, exercise, and mindfulness meditation. By gaining a greater understanding of how sleep works and why our body needs it, we are then empowered to have agency in valuing our sleep. You'll learn about the biological processes that govern sleep and how you'll be able to harness them to improve your sleep. After exploring how they affect your health and influence each other, I have provided some practical exercises to help you build healthy, sustainable practices within each area.

My own sleep journey has woven an incredible path through my life, from my own health to my partner's health to my profession. I am so thankful for the abundance of resources that enabled me to thoroughly explore and rewrite my own sleep story. In writing this book, I hope to share with you what I have learned over the years so that you can use it in whichever way best supports you.

I look forward to accompanying you on this journey as you explore *your* relationship to sleep. Whether you are interested in optimizing your sleep health or helping a loved one, I hope this book serves as a resource in your sleep journey and connects you to your healthiest self wherever you are in your life. Seldom do we give ourselves the permission to positively focus on sleeping, so the mere action of offering ourselves the space to acknowledge where we are right now in our sleep journeys can be foundational to building a sustainable sleep practice. It allows us to establish realistic goals and use what we're already doing well to bolster our efforts for change.

One final note: please be compassionate toward yourself in this process. When we explore and reflect on our own stories, we will inevitably uncover aspects of ourselves that make us uncomfortable in some way. Rather than avoid the discomfort, I encourage you to walk up to it and shake its hand. Your story is, after all, your bedside fellow.

—Daniel Jin Blum, PhD

"If sleep does not serve as an absolutely vital function, then it is the biggest mistake the evolutionary process has ever made."
—Dr. Allan Rechtschaffen, Sleep Research Pioneer[2]

PART ONE

SCIENCE OF SLEEP

Why do we sleep? With all the technological advances since the dawn of time, why do humans continue to spend a third of our lives, during the most vulnerable period of our circadian rhythm, unresponsive in bed? In this first section we explore these questions and begin to understand what's behind this realm that lies mostly outside of our consciousness.

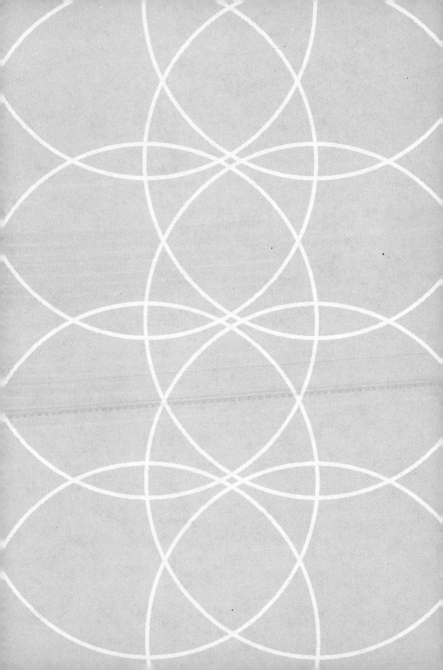

Chapter 1

WHY WE SLEEP

For most of us, sleep seems like a pretty simple process. We get into bed when we get tired at night, fall asleep, and wake up in the morning. We reap the rewards of sleep without realizing that sleep is *the* foundational element fueling our health. It's only when sleep gets knocked out of alignment that we suddenly realize how valuable it is; when we don't get enough, we feel more irritable and less focused. When we do, we feel happier and more energized. We are more resilient to stress, injury, and illness.

Part of the challenge is that many of the effects of sleep lie between barely perceptible to outside of conscious awareness. This is particularly so when the effects accumulate gradually over time. With the human capacity of adaptability, we tend to quickly shift our frame of reference to match our sleep-deprived states. While this is an incredibly helpful mechanism to get us through rough patches in the short-term, it can inadvertently perpetuate the perception that we can function on less sleep. The truth is that we can "function" on less sleep, but at levels far below our potential and for a much shorter time. With less sleep we can become quite good at functioning on autopilot, without engaging fully in life, and performing suboptimally.

I want to start with the "why" of sleep because this will help establish the purpose for sleep and its impact on our bodies and minds. Sleep serves an essential function in our lives and is not, as people thought for centuries, simply a maladaptive vestige of evolution. Contrary to old stereotypes that sleep is a waste of time, sleeping is actually quite a dynamic process that is a vital aspect of the body's daily renewal. While science is still uncovering the physiological reasons why we sleep, we do know that we need it to survive and will literally die without it.

Let's start with learning about the most crucial ways our bodies and minds benefit from sleep.

THE BODY

Our bodies are awe-inspiring machines; they grow, repair, and adapt to our surroundings without needing conscious thought. All of these amazing feats are enhanced and ultimately made possible by regular sleep. Just as regularly changing the oil in a car helps the engine run efficiently, sleeping gets the body to work at its efficient potential. Both will function without regular maintenance but with ever-decreasing efficiency—and both will inevitably stop working. Let's explore how your nights in bed provide the ideal situation to rest, renew, and repair your body.

Nourishes Cardiovascular Health

The heart, like all of the muscles in the body, requires "down time" to recover. Even though it continues to pump through the night, sufficient uninterrupted sleep provides a critical period of recovery. During this time, your heart can reduce its workload—measured in both heart rate and blood pressure—because it does not have to contend with gravity or with supplying oxygenated blood to multiple bodily processes that have slowed during sleep.

The acupuncturist for the Golden State Warriors once shared with me, "The heart only has so many beats." This simple insight, derived from his training in traditional Chinese medicine, stuck with me because it alludes to how the quality with which you treat your body affects the finite amount of time we have in this life. Rushing through life, stressed and unrested, can deplete your resources faster than they can recover. And, since the heart is the engine for your body, it is critically important to treat it with kindness. Nourishing your heart with high-quality sleep and exercise will encourage it to work harder for you and stretch every heartbeat to its fullest potential.

If, however, you work your heart tirelessly day and night, you expose yourself to an increased risk for hypertension and cardiovascular disease (the current leading cause of death for both men and women in the United States). Reducing your sleep even by a couple of hours per night can dramatically increase your risk for heart failure. Research shows that getting less than six hours of sleep per night can double the risk for having a stroke or heart attack.

When that number drops to five hours of sleep or less, your risk for a fatal heart attack is 45% greater compared to other adults who sleep at least seven hours.

Repairs Musculoskeletal System

Ever wonder why babies and kids need so much sleep? Sleep is essential to unlocking bone, muscle, and tissue development as well as repair. In this state of postural recumbence, our bones are no longer fighting the compression of gravity and are free to elongate, particularly during adolescence. The human body enhances this opportunity by releasing growth hormone to maximize this essential period of physical inactivity. Even when we are not in an active growth spurt, nighttime rest gives our muscles time to relax and repair. Everything in our bodies from our limbs to our hearts requires periods of sustained renewal. Without sufficient time to rest, muscles accumulate greater mileage, wear out faster, and leave us prone to injuries at a greater frequency and duration.

Flushes out Brain Toxins

One of the most recent findings on sleep functions is that sleep clears the brain of harmful toxins built up throughout the day. The brain is one of the most energy-intensive organs in the body for its size based on how much glucose it burns. As with any major processing center, running all day produces some residual waste that accumulates in the brain. When we sleep, our brains power down extraneous processes, which allows large swaths of neurons to rest.

Nightly rest for our brain cells helps maintain the sensitivity of the receptors that facilitate intercellular communication. Resting neurons also create space for cerebral spinal fluid to rush into the brain and flush out protein buildup. Similar to ocean tides washing a beach clear of footprints and debris, this fluid flows into the crevices of our brain and rinses out the toxins. This nightly process of waste removal was initially shown in mice and more recently confirmed in humans at UC Berkeley's Helen Wills Neuroscience Institute.[3]

When you are not getting enough sleep, you may begin to accumulate one particularly dangerous toxin called beta-amyloid. Singularly, beta-amyloid is merely a fragment of a larger protein used in the brain. However, this byproduct is particularly sticky and clumps together forming plaques in the brain, the same plaques that are strongly associated with Alzheimer's disease. Although the science is new, it appears that improving sleep reduces beta-amyloid plaques in the brain, which in essence could reduce one's risk for developing Alzheimer's disease later in life.

Boosts Immune Function

Have you ever found yourself getting sick after a big exam or project deadline? It's because your immune system has been significantly weakened from stress and lack of sleep. Proper sleep not only allows us to defend against oncoming illnesses, it also provides the right balance for building immunities for future infections. Uninterrupted sleep allows our bodies to balance the levels of immune defenses. When that process is interrupted, the first lines of defense—our ability to increase the inflammatory response to fight infection and the ability to recognize infected cells—are significantly compromised.

With even one hour of sleep loss each night for a week, our immune function can be suppressed by up to 44% of normal rates. If sleep loss continues unabated, as happens with many people with busy jobs or children, this deficit can jump to a 97% decrease in antibody production after just one month of partial sleep loss. It can be difficult to fathom that sleep could provide such a profound difference, but one of my clients experienced this firsthand.

A young female tech employee initially came to see me to see how she could fit more activities into her already packed schedule, which left insufficient time for her sleep. She noticed that she had been sick every month since moving to the Bay Area but was not entirely convinced that getting a little more sleep would significantly reduce these occurrences. Ambivalent about the impact but willing to try, she left my office. I did not hear from her for another few months, but when she returned, she relayed that she had not been sick once since increasing her sleep. I was also somewhat surprised at the immediate improvements, but it really exemplified this powerful connection between our sleep and our body's ability to stave off illness.

Acne, most commonly associate with our teenage years, is another infection that is exacerbated by frequently misaligned sleep patterns. Getting adequate sleep can boost our immune system and help decrease the duration and severity of outbreaks. The same acupuncturist friend said,

"When people ask for recommendations for facials I tell them to get some sleep!" The body requires a well-rested immune system to both effectively fight acne and keep your skin healthy.

Improves Metabolism

Just as sleep is critical for repairing muscles and building up the immune system, it is equally important in regulating our food intake. The hunger–satiety mechanisms in our bodies are normally regulated through the balance of two hormones: ghrelin and leptin. Ghrelin triggers our bodies to feel hungry and seek out nutrition. Once you find some food and put enough of it into your stomach, your fat cells then release leptin to tell you to stop eating. Ghrelin increases hunger, while leptin lessens hunger. When we get enough sleep, we don't worry about either, because they sync with our circadian schedules.

If our sleep gets off course, our hunger hormones get bumped out of rhythm along with it. This explains our tendency to reach for the donuts in the morning or why that pizza sounds so delicious at 2:00 a.m. First, your body will produce more ghrelin and cause you to want to seek out more food. With an increase in ghrelin activity, one would hope that your leptin response would follow suit. Unfortunately, it does just the opposite and delays the release of leptin. Together, this equates to a greater perceived need for food combined with continuing to eat beyond when your body normally tells you that you're full.

Your body's ability to regulate the incoming nutrients is

also tied to your sleep and circadian clock. Regular sleep stabilizes a large portion of your daily schedule and helps the pancreas coordinate the timing of your glucose and insulin responses. Glucose is the basic element of food that our bodies extract to fuel us during the day. Too much glucose production can lead to diabetes, so a well-rested pancreas will release insulin to balance out your blood sugar by encouraging cells to absorb glucose. The body has an amazing capacity to fine-tune on the fly, but a primary reason it works smoothly is because the schedule is predictable and the system is rested. The glucose response slows to repair itself during deep sleep along with your other muscles and organs. As morning approaches, it speeds up to prepare your body for the day. When you shorten your sleep, your body is not ready for an increase in glucose but your ghrelin starts telling you otherwise. This leads you to add more food to your diet, and thus more glucose into your system, which requires a larger insulin response. In brief spurts, your body adapts beautifully until you resume your healthy schedule. When sleep loss becomes chronic, your glucose and insulin responses can remain fatigued and malfunction, leading to more permanent deficits to the body's ability to self-regulate.

Sleep loss also triggers a similar response toward greater fat storage, which under chronic conditions of modern-day life can lead to excessive fat storage and weight gain. The chronic stress caused by continued sleep loss will compound this effect by breaking down muscles to replenish blood glucose levels and saving long-term energy (fat stores). This can quickly spiral downward because using muscle before fat increases the percentage of fat to muscle in your body *and* fat burns fewer calories than muscle. If left unchecked, this adds to the increase in calorie retention by converting more calories to fat, which burns fewer calories, leaving additional unused calories around to convert into fat.

As these appetite-related processes begin to spiral downward, many people seek refuge in the power of the brain—our willpower, our ability to think rationally and make good choices—to help turn things around. Our brains help us identify an issue, seek out the etiology, and motivate us toward change. As with all of the other organs, the brain functions optimally with regular, sufficient rest, but it is also very resilient in the face of adversity. However, eventually it will succumb to the effects of chronic sleep loss and its deteriorating functioning will contribute to the dietary downward spiral. As your body begins to have a greater propensity for craving more calories, storing more of them as fat, and burning them at a slower rate, your brain's ability to resist unhealthy foods, particularly those that contain refined carbohydrates and sugars, is compromised. The part of your brain responsible for behavioral inhibition, the prefrontal cortex, begins to have lapses in judgment with inadequate rest. Meanwhile, the physiological stress of sleep loss will start a chain reaction that increases levels of neuropeptide Y, a chemical that increases your *desire* for carbs. As you can see, once the stress of chronic sleep loss takes effect, it sets in motion a chain of many processes that perpetuate the cycle.

THE MIND

While flushing out toxins helps the physical health of the brain, the application of thought and emotion reflects the health of the more ethereal mind. It's in the mind where we most immediately notice when we don't sleep well the night before. Sleep influences the ability of the brain to regulate our emotions, harness our concentration, access memories, and engage in positive relationships.

Regulates Emotions

Sleep is crucial for replenishing neurotransmitters that help to understand, express, and regulate emotions. These amazing benefits typically go unnoticed when you're getting enough sleep. It's when you get one or more short or fragmented nights that you might notice an increase in your irritability and a shorter fuse. It may manifest as an exasperated sigh when your child spills his bowl of food all over the floor or a biting comment that leaps out of your mouth when your partner mentions that he or she got a parking ticket.

The increased tendency to *react* when you're sleep deprived is also seen in functional magnetic resonance imaging brain scans. Studies that utilize this specialized equipment show that the amygdala, part of our brain's emotional control center, becomes significantly more activated when we are short of sleep. Normally, our logical center, the prefrontal cortex, will assess the situation and help us calm down if the amygdala becomes overactive. The prefrontal cortex is a newer section of the brain that has evolved to help us discern real threats from perceived ones. If your amygdala warns your prefrontal cortex that something is scratching at your door, your prefrontal cortex will assess if the sound is simply your cat wanting to come back in (rather than an intruder or unknown threat) and will signal your body to calm down. However, without enough sleep, the amygdala chooses to leave the prefrontal cortex out of the decision-making process. With the emotional brain in charge, it will signal the fight or flight system in an older part of the brain, to get you ready to react quickly to real danger—but more often than not the threat is a perceived danger, not a real one.

Once you get your sleep back on track, your emotional brain will become less active and will resume communication with the logical brain to help assess experiences. Your mood will improve and things will feel less anxiety-provoking as you regularly rest and reset your brain. When sleep debt begins to accumulate again without replenishment, your mood will stay in this zone of increased vigilance.

Relieves Stress

When you don't get enough sleep, your stress-response system, also called the *sympathetic nervous system* or fight or flight system, is activated. This system works best when stressors are short-lived. It increases your heart rate and blood flow to your muscles, focuses your senses on your surroundings, and tenses your muscles for action. While this vigilant state prepares you to either fight off an attacker or run away, it is not great for thinking or reasoning because internal resources have been temporarily diverted to improve reactivity. Once you reach safety, your body engages the parasympathetic nervous system to relax your body and return to equilibrium.

Your stress response, while incredibly handy in acute situations, alters your perceptions of your environment. During this state of heightened vigilance, studies have found that individuals deprived of sleep over one night were significantly more reactive to negatively themed photos (e.g., pictures of snakes or injuries) compared to well-slept participants. This reactivity subsequently affects memory. The well-slept participants remembered both the positive- and negative-themed images with equal frequency, while the sleep-deprived individuals remembered the negative-themed images equally well, but did not remember as many of the positive images.

Overall, the increased emotional reactivity caused by stress is incredibly adaptive because it optimizes your body and mind for survival. If the stress becomes chronic, as seen in accumulated sleep debt, the heightened emotional reactivity can quickly contribute to the development of an anxiety or mood disorder. A study at a hospital in Norway found that people with insomnia were twenty times more likely to develop panic disorder, a type of anxiety disorder. This same study also found that sleep-deprived people were five times as likely to develop depression compared to well-slept individuals. The nature of this relationship between insomnia and psychiatric disorders has also been shown to be predictive, in that insomnia was a reliable predictor of the onset of depression or anxiety. Coupled with the unfortunate "normalcy" of this kind of perpetual sleep loss of one or two hours per night, it's easy to see why healthy sleep is essential in both preventing and alleviating anxious and depressive symptoms.

Increases Concentration

Related to fluctuations in mood, difficulties with concentration are also common side effects of inadequate sleep. Proper rest helps maintain lower levels of physiological stress and leaves our mental reservoirs fully stocked to divert to the task at hand. As sleep loss begins to creep in, mental reserves begin to leak out to attend to the ambient stress caused by feeling tired. Our bodies are equipped to handle this in small amounts and may only show minor blips in processing power. With habitual drainage, one's mental reserves shrink alongside the ability to concentrate both in terms of acuity and duration.

Obtaining high-quality sleep also influences our ability to focus our attention. Where some people with chronic sleep deprivation respond with depressive or anxious symptoms, others begin to exhibit core symptoms of attention deficit/hyperactivity disorder (ADHD). A recent study at Duke University showed that up to 95% of obstructive sleep apnea clients experienced attentional deficits. This includes difficulties with concentration, behavioral inhibition, and hyperactivity. Additionally, when sleep issues were treated in participants with ADHD, they experienced significant improvements in concentration and hyperactivity.

Enhances Learning & Memory

As we learn new skills and experience novel situations during the day, getting enough sleep at night provides the setting to categorize, reorganize, and store this information efficiently for later use. The kinds of information we acquire vary considerably, from typing on your computer to understanding your connection to a greater whole. We'll learn more about the relationship between the type of information we learn and the different stages of sleep in the next chapter.

As your brain balances sleep needs based on the type of informational input, it begins to streamline the information for ease of retrieval by activating different parts of the brain than those used during the learning phase. While you are sleeping, the brain reorganizes the information learned from the areas that specialize in receiving external stimuli and moves it to areas that specialize in the desired output of the memories. For example, when you begin to learn how to type, the areas of the brain that help with spatial recognition in the parietal lobe would activate while learning and practicing the task. At the beginning, typing is challenging. It takes effort and concentration to learn the location of the keys and coordinate your fingers to tap them in the desired sequence. But, each time you fall asleep following a practice session, your brain will gradually shift the storage of this new information to sections of the prefrontal cortex that control motor movements. Eventually, this subtle change automates this process by reducing the need to think about typing and allowing the motor cortex to run the typing programs in the background, thus increasing the speed and accuracy of your typing.

Cultivates Positive Relationships

Lastly, and maybe most important, sleep affects how we interact with others. Consistently healthy sleep allows us to see where others are coming from more often and let more things roll off our backs. It allows us to calm down more quickly when we become upset and experience joy more frequently. It cultivates our compassion, humor, and connectedness. Conversely, sleep debt quickens our temper and makes us more prone to argument. Adding this stressor to our bodies consumes more energy and attention and leaves us vulnerable to emotional reactivity instead of intentionally choosing our responses. It narrows our worldview and even impairs our ability to accurately read facial expressions and social cues.

In addition, sleep-deprived individuals have difficulties discerning the differences between friendly and threatening facial expressions. Due to this difficulty, people will tend to misinterpret neutral and friendly expressions as threatening. Although it is adaptive to quickly perceive threats to protect ourselves in the short-term, it can lead to frequent miscommunications with our partners, friends, and families. Interpreting more interactions as threatening can even lead to retreating more from the world. And with that isolation comes increased loneliness simply from neglecting our sleep.

When we finally get some sleep, particularly REM (rapid

eye movement) sleep, our emotional ship begins to right itself. We feel more rested, energetic, and social, all of which help to reconnect us with those we care about.

PUTTING IT ALL TOGETHER

From the cellular to the interpersonal level, sleep is the foundation of our health and one of the cornerstones of living well. The intention of this chapter is that if we build our awareness around sleep health, we become more incentivized to prioritize sleep amid the numerous demands that vie for our time and attention. The countless hours we spend studying for school, pursuing our craft, or practicing a hobby pale in comparison to the time we actually sleep. Sleep enhances all of these activities, yet it is often the first item we sacrifice when we feel busy or overwhelmed.

Getting enough sleep will help us operate at our highest potentials across several domains. And in a world that's demanding us to perform ever more highly, getting the proper sleep can help us maximize our ability to feel better, work smarter, and become more resilient.

Chapter 2

HOW SLEEP WORKS

Now that we know what sleep does for us, let's understand how sleep actually works. Prior to brain imaging technology, which allows researchers to peek inside the sleeping brain, the medical field conceived sleep as an "intermediary step between life and death," a static process that wasn't much different than being in a coma or vegetative state. As the field of sleep medicine began to gain traction in the latter half of the twentieth century, we discovered it was quite the contrary, that our sleep was incredibly complex and dynamic, made up of multiple biological systems that worked in concert with each other.

In this chapter we will explore these systems and how they interact to produce healthy sleep, which is defined here as both optimal quantity and high quality. The quantity refers to the amount of sleep we get per night: the ideal amount for your age and your body to feel rested. The quality refers to the restorative properties of sleep we get throughout the night: the ideal proportion of each stage of sleep to perform well. Sleep quality is better related than quantity to improved measures of health, well-being and performance. While there's a tendency to focus on the sleep quantity, it's important to remember that both are critical and one is not sufficient on its own.

As a forewarning, this is perhaps the most scientifically dense part of this book. For some, the prospect of digging into the science may sound exciting, while others may feel themselves already starting to yawn. In either case, you may want to consider taking your time to digest this chapter. Yes, it is a lot to wade through, but it serves as an important first step.

With my clients, I always start with the science because it helps us gain a greater understanding of how sleep works. By doing so, it demystifies the black box of sleep and empowers us to have agency in identifying and changing unhealthy sleep. Additionally, understanding the biological mechanisms that underlie our sleeping and waking states will also provide the requisite rationale that informs the strategies that we will eventually employ.

If it helps, think about this as your sleep manual. You're learning about the basic components, how the different mechanisms function, and what the different levers are. Once you have a good grasp, you can operate your sleep in the way it was designed.

SLEEP AMOUNT

Whenever someone learns that I'm a sleep psychologist, inevitably, the first question I get is, "So, how much sleep do I *really* need?" Usually followed by "I heard" or "I read." The old adage that "everyone needs eight hours of sleep" is gradually being replaced with more scientific recommendations based on age and individual variability. Some of you must be thinking, "I knew it! I run fine on five hours a night," or know someone who would feel justified. But before you get too excited at the prospect, it turns out that 95% of adults need between 7 and 9 hours to function at their best. And even then, half of the remaining 5% need more. So that leaves less than 2.5% of the population that needs less than the recommended amount. You may be in that group, but, statistically speaking, it's very unlikely.

Recommended Sleep

The amount of sleep that we need, as adults, meaning that we are allowing our bodies and minds to fully recharge, is between 7 and 9 hours. As infants we need the most amount of sleep, anywhere from 14 to 17 hours. This gradually decreases to 8 to 10 hours by adolescence and eventually stabilizes around 7 to 9 hours through adulthood. The following graphic provides general guidelines by the National Sleep Foundation and is based on more than two years of research. It gives you a good idea of where your personal ideal amount of sleep lies and is a great place to start.

What's your recommended amount?

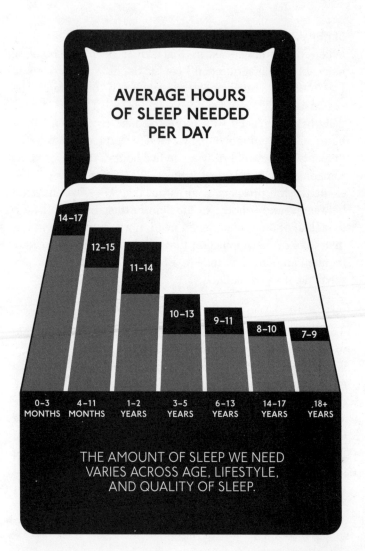

AVERAGE HOURS
OF SLEEP NEEDED
PER DAY

14–17

12–15

11–14

10–13

9–11

8–10

7–9

| 0–3 MONTHS | 4–11 MONTHS | 1–2 YEARS | 3–5 YEARS | 6–13 YEARS | 14–17 YEARS | 18+ YEARS |

THE AMOUNT OF SLEEP WE NEED
VARIES ACROSS AGE, LIFESTYLE,
AND QUALITY OF SLEEP.

Once you find your sleep range, you can begin to tinker with your personal ideal because your optimal sleep duration ultimately comes down to your subjective experience: how much sleep do you need to feel at your best in your current life circumstances? Some people feel at their cognitive and physical peaks after consistently getting 9 hours of sleep per night while others feel 7 hours is optimal. Elite athletes generally need one additional hour of sleep compared to same-aged peers. Or if you catch a cold, temporarily increasing your sleep helps your body rest and recover.

As you begin to collect your own sleep data in Chapter 3, you can start to notice the relationship between how much you sleep at night and how you feel during the day. Remember, it's about finding what's optimal for you to function at your best.

SLEEP CYCLES

Much of our day-to-day lives revolve around daily pulses called *circadian rhythms*. Circadian comes from the Latin words *circa* and *diem,* which roughly translates to "approximately one day," and describes the body's daily internal timer for sleepiness and alertness. Our sleep cycles are a major part of our circadian rhythms. The interplay between sleep and circadian rhythms provides the broad framework for sleep and wakefulness. It illuminates the fluctuations of feeling alert or sleepy over the course of a day and lays the foundation for timing our sleep-wake cycles with our natural rhythms.

Nested within each day-long circadian period are shorter

cycles called *ultradian* cycles. They are much shorter in duration, last anywhere from 70 to 120 minutes, and repeat several times over the course of a day. Sleep is made up of these ultradian cycles that rhythmically pulse throughout the night.

So an evening's rest is actually composed of several ultradian sleep cycles, with each cycle moving through four distinct stages: light sleep, unequivocal sleep, deep sleep, and REM, or rapid eye movement. Each stage serves its own unique purpose. The first three stages comprise the majority, or up to 80%, of our sleep. As we progress into each stage, several processes are occurring: our brain waves become slower and more synchronized, our breathing and heart rate eases, and our senses dim, making us harder to arouse.

First Stage: Light Sleep

The first stage is called light sleep, or N1, and encompasses the transition between being awake and entering sleep. N1 serves as a primer for our bodies and minds to sleep and makes up only around 5 to 10% of our total sleep. It is the lightest stage of sleep, so ambient noise or hearing one's name called can jog someone out of this state and back into waking life. This is also the stage where people may experience a sudden feeling of falling and jerk themselves awake. This sensation, known as *hypnic myoclonia* or more commonly as "sleep starts," can be a startling experience but is brief and quite common.

Second Stage: Unequivocal Sleep

After spending a few minutes in light sleep, our brains fully transition into sleep mode by the time we reach stage two, or N2. Though still considered a type of light sleep, our arousal threshold increases, making it harder to wake us up and, thus, protecting our journey into slumber. This stage is characterized by distinct bursts of brain activity, called sleep spindles and K-complexes, which are key for language acquisition and motor memory consolidation. Adults spend the most time in this stage, from 45% to 55% each night.

Third Stage: Deep Sleep

The third stage, or N3, is the deepest stage of sleep. This is when your brain waves appear as slow rhythmic delta waves on an electroencephalogram (EEG). It is frequently referred to as slow-wave sleep (SWS) or delta sleep. N3 is the most difficult from which to rouse someone, so it is also aptly called deep sleep or restorative sleep. Trying to wake someone from this stage is often met with grogginess, not to mention significant grumpiness. Deep sleep occurs predominantly during the first third of the night and decreases with each subsequent ultradian sleep cycle. N3 has been associated with improving certain types of memories but is best known for its association with the growth and repair of body tissue, muscle, and bone. The timing of slow wave sleep has been shown to work in concert with the body's natural cycle of releasing growth hormones typically around 1:00 a.m. to 2:00 a.m., but also during daytime naps if someone has been deprived of deep sleep the night before. Overall, the healthy adult will only spend 10% to 20% of his or her slumber in deep sleep.

It is important to note that we do not immediately go into REM stage right after our deep sleep. Our sleep must cycle back through unequivocal and light stages of sleep, though at a faster rate. So we climb in and out of this light-deep-light sleep trough—N1 to N2 to N3 to N2 to N1— before we enter into the first REM stage.

Last Stage: REM

REM is the last stage of sleep before you begin a new ultra-dian cycle and is where vivid cinematic and imaginative dreams typically occur. Flying through space, exploring new cities, or running away from danger are some of the exciting backdrops that occupy your mind while your body rests. As you probably surmised, REM sleep is characterized by rapid eye movements during sleep. Normal rapid movements during sleep sounds counterintuitive to the purpose of rest, which is also why it is referred to as paradoxical sleep. Due to the active nature of such dreams, your body temporarily paralyzes you, a condition known as muscle *atonia,* to ensure that you're not actually running around. At the beginning of the night, your REM stages are quite brief, lasting only a few minutes. This gradually shifts during the night as the duration of each REM period steadily lengthens with every subsequent cycle.

REM comprises the second greatest proportion of sleep, and research indicates that it serves a critical role in consolidating knowledge learned during the previous day. It makes up as high as 50% of a given night of sleep during infancy and slowly decreases to around 20 to 25% in adulthood. Adolescents and college students I've worked with often find this piece of information quite interesting because it is contrary to the well-known practice of "pulling an all-nighter." The ancient tradition of "cramming" facts into your head before an exam relies on the hope that the brain is like a bucket that you stuff information into all night. Such students believe the longer you are awake to add in information, the more you will have access to the following day. In actuality, without enough sleep, your brain will act more like a sieve. The human brain has an amazing capacity to store information but still requires sleep to properly integrate it into memory. Getting at least four full REM cycles of sleep after studying will help you store that knowledge so you can effectively retrieve it the next day. If we get woken up at any of these stages, once we fall back asleep, we have to go back through all the stages that precede it, though at a much faster rate.

Now that we understand what makes up the components of sleep, let's explore the mechanisms that allow us to fall and stay asleep.

SLEEP MECHANISMS

A lot of people think sleep is an on/off switch, but anyone who has struggled to fall asleep knows it's not that easy. Sleep is actually governed by an intricate interaction between three different mechanisms: the homeostatic sleep drive, the circadian wake drive, and the arousal system. Think about these processes as levers that help us operate our sleep.

The first two processes, sleep and wake, are the primary drivers that regulate our sleep. They help to keep us alert during the day and determine when we go to bed, when we wake up, and when we might need a nap. In the case of an emergency, our arousal system, or the third process, serves as a safety mechanism and will override the first two to wake us up. It's like sleep's version of an emergency brake. With that, let's pop open the hood and get a better sense of how each one of these works.

Sleep Drive

Our homeostatic sleep drive, or process S, acts as our sleep-iness fuel gage, telling us when we have enough to function well during the day or when we need to fill up. As the day continues, our need for sleep steadily increases. Our *sleep homeostat* keeps running tabs on how much sleep we've used and will let us know when it's time to put away that last email or cocktail and get to sleep. The need for sleep is at its highest when our eyes are drooping and all that's running through our mind is "I'm so sleepy." If you have ever stayed up late or pulled an all-nighter, that feeling of extreme fatigue is your homeostatic sleep drive demanding that you get some sleep. Once we finally get enough rest, our need for sleep returns to its lowest point and our tank is full.

As a side note, we may still feel a bit groggy after we wake up from a full night of sleep. This natural phenomenon is very common and known as *sleep inertia*. It usually wears off after 5 to 60 minutes. If the grogginess persists for several hours, it could be a sign that you need a tune-up. Often, we override our bodies' natural cue to get rest by drinking coffee or other artificial stimulants to stay awake. We'll discuss the implications of caffeine in our sleep quality in Chapter 9.

Influence of Adenosine

But how does our *sleep homeostat* work? What is the biological mechanism behind it? The most consistent chemical proxy for our sleep drive is associated with the accumulation of adenosine, which is part of adenosine triphosphate (ATP) or the molecular structure of stored energy. When we actively use our brains during the day and extract energy for ATP, the byproduct of this use, adenosine, accumulates faster than our brains can get rid of it. As the levels of adenosine continue to rise, they begin to block the alerting signals in our brain that are keeping us alert during the day, thus making us feel sleepier. Once we fall asleep at night, our brains requires less energy so the rate of adenosine accumulation slows down. This period of rest then allows the enzymes that scrub adenosine from our brains to quickly break it down so we can wake up in the morning without feeling too groggy.

If adenosine is slowly making us increasingly sleepier throughout the day, you may be wondering how we can stay alert and focused. Why don't our energy levels steadily drain like a battery from dawn to dusk? The human body has adapted beautifully to this challenge by balancing your sleep drive with another amazing mechanism called the circadian process to keep you relatively alert until just before you sleep.

Wake Drive

To offset our sleep drive, our bodies naturally produce an alerting signal that keeps us active and functioning during the day. This is known as the circadian wake drive, or process C, which is influenced by our internal clock and closely mirrors the rhythm of the homeostatic sleep drive.

The wake drive follows a wave: it rises in the morning to wake us up, dips slightly mid-day, boosts right before bedtime, drops sharply to help us fall asleep, continues to drop to help us stay asleep, and then begins to rise again a few hours before we wake up. So it makes sense that, as adults, we generally feel sleepiest in the early morning between 1:00 a.m. and 4:00 a.m. and then again in the early afternoon between 1:00 p.m. to 3:00 p.m. The post-lunch drowsiness is actually a natural dip in our circadian pulse and not just the product of boring meetings. Conversely, we often feel the most alert shortly after awakening and again just before bedtime between 6:00 p.m. to 9:00 p.m. The evening burst is usually followed by a quick drop in energy, which makes it ideal for falling asleep if we time it correctly. Our ability to sleep during the night and feel alert during the day works best when we are able to sync these two processes together.

While these two processes are conceptualized as independent systems, they dynamically influence each other.

This explains why we can be both sleepy and wired at the same time. For example, you have a late night working on a presentation and don't get to bed until midnight; you don't get a full night's rest, so your sleep drive is still high. When your alarm clock goes off in the morning, you're obviously tired because you didn't get enough sleep. But since your circadian wake drive is also high, you're able to wake up and give your presentation. If your sleep and wake drives didn't operate independently, then your sleep drive would be overriding your wakefulness and you would get progressively sleepier during your own presentation.

Influence of Circadian Rhythm & Light

Our master circadian, or internal, clocks govern our wake drive, which is actually quite malleable and moves slightly longer than the 24-hour day. The full-length of most adults' circadian clocks stretches out to 24.2-hours. This means that instead of synchronizing perfectly with every full rotation of the earth, an adult's sleep-wake cycle naturally resets just past the 24-hour mark each day. That little fraction of time may seem minute to some, but if you let this natural clock run your life, you would naturally go to bed and wake up 10 minutes later each day. If you think that sounds disruptive, adolescents have it even worse. Not only do they need more sleep (8–10 hours), their circadian rhythm ticks on a 24.4-hour cycle, shifting their bed and wake times forward as much as 27 minutes per day! That's more than 3 hours in a week, or the equivalent of moving across three time zones. As you could imagine, adhering just to your circadian schedule could wreak havoc on your ability to sync up to your work, school, and social engagements.

So how do we maintain our regular schedules? Fortunately, the external environment is enormously helpful in getting us to make both major and minor adjustments to realign us to regular daytime schedules. These external circadian cues are called *zeitgebers,* or time-givers in German, and serve as helpful reminders throughout the day that aide in aligning one's internal clock with the environment. Notable zeitgebers include light, social obligations, meals, exercise, and ambient temperature. Of these, light is the most important and sets the pace for our circadian wake drive.

Light has the single strongest influence on our internal clock. Inside the brain, this clock is primarily regulated by the suprachiasmatic nucleus (SCN), a small bundle of nerves located in the hypothalamus just behind your eyes. Once the sun sets and light, particularly short blue-wave light, stops entering the eye, this circadian timekeeper signals the pineal gland to begin releasing melatonin, a sleep-promoting hormone in diurnal animals. As ambient darkness deepens, melatonin continues to rise and communicates with the rest of the body to increase relaxation, decrease core body temperature, and optimize body and mind for slumber. It has a gradual effect on the body and reaches its peak powers around 2:00 a.m. to 5:00 a.m., coinciding with one of our major sleep valleys. Our body metabolizes and eliminates it during the night so it is normally gone when the sun rises in the morning.

Influence of Cortisol & Melatonin

When light stimulates our internal clock, it signals to the brain to release hormones to help us wake up (cortisol), or fall asleep (melatonin). When light streams into one's eyes first thing in the morning, it stimulates the SCN, which tells the body that it's time to wake up. The circadian pacemaker signals the adrenal glands to release additional cortisol, which then signals the body to increase alertness, continue to raise body temperature, and get the organs and muscles ready for the day. After the additional burst in the morning, cortisol levels steadily drop over the course of the day. When the sun sets in the evening and you stop receiving light into your eyes, your master clock then signals your pineal gland to start releasing melatonin. As our melatonin levels rise over the course of several hours, our cortisol levels continue to drop, which helps us power down for the evening and prepare for sleep. After peaking in the early morning, melatonin levels steadily drop as we sleep and our cortisol levels rise to help prepare the body to wake up and start the day. As the sun starts rising, melatonin levels drop, cortisol begins rising. It's really quite amazing how our bodies coordinate this complex motion outside of conscious awareness every day simply with the natural shifts of light and darkness.

However, this wonderfully beneficial sensitivity to this zeitgeber can also delay our ability to wind down at night if light is introduced too late into the evening or too early in the morning. Setting our internal clocks to the regular cycle of the sun worked well up through the pre-Industrial

Revolution era when people typically rose with the sun and slept after it set. The introduction of artificial light was a marvelous technological advancement and had a profound effect on productivity; unfortunately, this new ability to generate continuous light on demand also had an unfortunate effect on sleep.

Due to the relatively new invention of electricity, our brains have still not had sufficient time to differentiate between artificial light and sunlight. The circadian timekeeper responds similarly to both artificial light and sunlight and can delay the release of melatonin in the continued presence of either. This causes a chain reaction by postponing the body's normal process of getting ready for sleep—until we finally turn off our TVs, computers, smartphones, and so on. The light from these devices is strong enough to hold up our sleep schedule and can make it difficult to fall asleep. Among cultures and subpopulations where electricity is scarce or nonexistent, sleep follows the more natural cycles of night and day, even among adolescents whose biological propensities for sleep are shifted. While a renunciation of all digital devices is a bit extreme, intentionally reducing our usage of electronics after sunset is a positive behavior to incorporate into any healthy sleep practice.

Arousal System
If the homeostatic sleep drive and circadian wake drive are the primary processes that govern our sleep, it's the arousal system, or process W, that can override them both. This is known as the "warning system" or "wake system" and can

override the other two sleep rhythms if you are in danger. For example, if the fire alarm goes off in the middle of the night, your arousal system will wake you up and get you out of bed to safety. It is quite an adaptive process because no matter how dark or how sleepy you feel, this system will temporarily override your sleep and keep you alert until you reach safety. Once the danger has subsided, the arousal system will calm down and sleep can return. The only issue arises when this system is continually activated through chronic stress. Pressures from work, relationships, and life may not cause the same jolt of adrenaline. However, this continual activation can keep the system elevated throughout the day and into the night, which can disrupt your ability to relax and fall asleep at bedtime. If stress from any domain can increase the arousal system, it may sound impossible to ever tamp it down and get consistent sleep. Fortunately, the arousal system is incredibly responsive to mindfulness and relaxation practices. If you can incorporate mindfulness practices into your regular routine, you will be able to not only calm your arousal system, but anticipate when you may need a few extra minutes to reset during a stressful day.

PUTTING IT ALL TOGETHER

Congratulations, you finished the Science of Sleep 101! Learning why we sleep and how sleep works is no small feat. You may not feel that you've completely grasped all the concepts, and that's okay. As we look at your sleep in the upcoming chapters, these systems will start to make more sense and, as with any good guide, you can always refer back to this section to help clarify points of confusion.

"Knowing yourself is the beginning of all wisdom."
—Aristotle [4]

PART TWO

YOUR SLEEP

Let's now shift the focus from the external information on sleep medicine to the internal reflection of your sleep. This section provides guidance on how to track your sleep and break down the unique aspects of your life—different thoughts, emotions, and behaviors—that impact your sleep story. By gaining a clearer picture of your current sleep patterns and a thoughtful examination of your sleep narrative, we can identify how to optimize your sleep.

Chapter 3

SLEEP ASSESSMENT

Many of us know that we want more sleep, but how do we know how much more we need? As someone who tends to think linearly, I find that getting a clearer picture of current sleep patterns and establishing baseline levels of sleep is an important first step toward changing one's sleep patterns. A thoughtful examination of our stories and patterns surrounding sleep will help us decide the best course of action.

To help you get a better understanding of the current state of your sleep, this chapter provides tools to track your sleep. The data you collect can help illuminate areas where you can identify unhealthy sleep patterns and intervene with different strategies to improve them.

TRACKING YOUR SLEEP

The small act of recording your sleep times is a step toward prioritizing your health and well-being. How so? Each day you recount your sleep is another incremental step toward bringing sleep into your sphere of consciousness. And as your awareness builds, your drive to engage in sleep-promoting behaviors grows with it. The consistent tracking also provides valuable insights into how your sleep schedule fluctuates from day to day and week to week, surfacing patterns that you might not have noticed.

Sleep Log

As a method for self-tracking your sleep, the sleep log is an effective strategy for illuminating self-reported sleep-related practices. It is cheap, simple, and quick to use. Its simplicity and reliability has facilitated its ubiquitous use in research and clinical care, which makes it the "gold standard" tool for tracking sleep among clinicians.

The work of maintaining a sleep log, while simple, can be a potential barrier for people starting an intentional sleep practice. Life can at times feel oppressively busy, even frenetic. Adding one more item to the to-do list may not sound appetizing, especially when it already feels as though you don't have enough time to do everything you want, hence the sleep loss! Fortunately, tracking your sleep takes less than a minute and provides valuable information to help improve your sleep.

Once you prioritize your sleep, you will find that you will accomplish your daily activities in shorter amounts of time and of equal or better quality. This small step of only 30 seconds will at the very least provide a detailed picture of your sleep patterns. Being specific about your intention of completing the diary will increase the likelihood that you follow through.

Getting Started

To start mapping out your sleep, you can find several free examples of sleep diaries online. For the purposes of this book, I have included a template based on the Consensus Sleep Diary, which was developed by a team of sleep researchers and clinicians. It is the standard format used in research and clinical applications and can be customized based on one's needs. I prefer to use this format for its simplicity and because it captures the essential domains to help you sleep.

When adding a new entry to your sleep log, it is best to fill it out shortly after you wake up in the morning. Your memory of the previous night's sleep is often at its best at that time and you won't have to think about completing it later in your day. At the UC Berkeley Sleep Lab, I have clients pick a consistent time each morning and pick a location where they will keep the diary, for example, *7:30 a.m., on my bedroom desk.* Once a client sets their schedule, I have them visualize themselves putting the sleep log on the desk and then completing it in the morning. This last step is important because it begins to groove the neuropathways in the brain related to completing your intention.

Each line is fairly self-explanatory, and you can use the example in the second column as a reference for how to complete each line. However, make sure to read each item carefully to ensure that you're tracking your sleep accurately. I've provided explanations of each category for you to reference when filling it out the first few times:

Bed Time (BT)

Bed Time is the time that you physically get into bed. For some people, this is the same time that they try to fall asleep but for many of us, we get into bed and read or use one of a variety of devices before actually trying to fall asleep. I had one client tell me that her bed time was 11:00 p.m., but when I asked her what she was doing in the hour before, she told me that she was watching TV in bed from 9:00 p.m. onward. Going through each line of the diary with her was crucial because it helped her understand this difference.

Lights Out (LO)

Lights Out is the moment that you turn everything off (lights, devices, etc.) and try to fall asleep. If this is the same as your Bed Time, simply put the same time again. However, if you are poking around on your device for an hour before finally putting it down, make sure to record that moment as the time you turned your Lights Out.

Sleep Onset Latency (SOL)

Sleep Onset Latency is the technical term for how long it takes you to fall asleep. The timer begins when you start actually trying to fall asleep (i.e., when you get into bed and after Lights Out) and lasts until you begin sleeping. Turning off all the lights includes screens as well, such as TVs, laptops, tablets, and smartphones. This is an important distinction because so many of us will turn off lamps or overhead lights but continue to receive light from screens. Remember, the timer starts when *all* of your light sources are off. It can be difficult to pinpoint the exact moment we fall asleep because we experience brief retrograde amnesia (a loss of memory for prior events) at that moment of sleep. However, for the purposes of tracking your own sleep, your best guess is sufficient.

Wake After Sleep Onset (WASO)

Wake After Sleep Onset represents the total amount of time you spent awake when you woke up during the night after you initially fell asleep. For example, if you fell asleep at 10:00 p.m. and woke up twice (once for 10 minutes and the other time for 15 minutes) before you finally get out of your bed in the morning, you would write the sum of those values under WASO, in this case 25 minutes.

It is important to record the total duration of your nighttime awakenings because it will affect both how useful your sleep was and your total sleep time. Many people wake up once or twice per night for a few minutes or less each time. As long as each episode is less than 5–10 minutes, it should not have too much of a detrimental effect on your sleep. However, if you wake up more often or for longer periods of time (greater than 30 minutes per night), it will begin to negatively impact your sleep and subsequently your day.

When people say they "sleep eight hours a night" it often means that they *allocate* eight hours for sleep every night. When you begin to factor in when they turned off their lights, how long it took them to fall asleep, and how long they were awake during the middle of the night, eight hours of sleep shrinks quickly. Your body can become accustomed to a fragmented sleep schedule as well so teasing this out across the course of a week will help you determine if lying awake in bed was an aberration or a recurring issue.

Wake Time (WT)
Wake Time is recorded as the last time you awoke before getting out of bed to start your day. If you're one of the many people who use the snooze button two to three times before getting out of bed, record the time you finally wake up after you stop snoozing your alarm clock.

Rise Time (RT)
Rise Time is when you finally get out of your bed for the day. If you get up within a few minutes of awakening, then

this should be similar to your WT. However, if you tend to lounge in bed looking at your phone, reading, or simply enjoying the morning, your RT will be later than your wake time.

Time In Bed (TIB)

Time In Bed represents the total amount of time you spent in your bed. Calculating how much time you spend in bed helps shed light on how much time you're using your bed for activities other than sleep or sex (e.g., homework, talking on the phone, eating, watching TV, etc.). Our beds or bedrooms can sometimes be the only personal space we have for periods of our lives, so it can be tempting to use it as an office or lounge. However, the more we use the bed for these reasons, the more our bodies and minds become accustomed to being awake in bed, and the harder it becomes to fall asleep when we want to.

To find your TIB for any given day, simply determine the length of time you spent in bed between the time you got into bed at night (BT) until you finally got out of bed in the morning (RT). For example, if you got into bed at 9:00 p.m. and out of bed the next morning at 8:00 a.m., your TIB for that night would be 11 hours. However, if you get out of bed for a significant amount of time during the night for any reason or spend more than a few minutes out of bed, make sure to subtract that time from your total. For example, if you left your bed twice during the night for 30 minutes each time, your TIB would be 10 hours instead of 11.

Total Sleep Time (TST)

Total Sleep Time is the total amount of time you spent actually sleeping. In the context of a sleep log, this provides more precision than the typical estimate that people generally use: "I went to bed at 11:00 p.m. and got up at 7:00 a.m., so I got 8 hours of sleep." Unless you fall asleep immediately upon hitting the bed, which is not the norm and would indicate a severe sleep deficiency, the amount you actually slept (TST) is often shorter than the time you spent in bed (TIB).

First, calculate the time difference between when you tried to fall asleep (LO) and your final awakening (WT). Once you have this number, subtract how long it took you to fall asleep (SOL) and how long you were awake at night (WASO). This value is your TST. In the example listed in the sleep log provided, the difference between when this person tried to fall asleep (LO: 10:15 p.m.) and his final awakening (WT: 7:30 a.m.) was 9 hours 15 minutes. You would then subtract how long it took to fall asleep (SOL; 15 min) as well as how long he was awake during the night (WASO; 20 min), leaving you with a total sleep time (TST) of 8 hours 40 minutes.

This number can be very helpful early on in illuminating that "sleeping for 8 hours" actually means that you need to be in bed trying to fall asleep at least 8.5 hours before your desired wakening for example. Knowing your TST will also help you understand how efficient your sleep is and can thus inform additional changes you can employ to improve your sleep.

Sleep Efficiency (SE)

Sleep Efficiency is a great tool to help you determine if your ability to fall asleep is working effectively. While we cannot directly apply effort to falling asleep, we can improve our sleep by changing some of the domains related to sleeping (creating separation between sleep and work, bright lights, stressors, etc.). If you have ever tried to concentrate on falling asleep you probably experienced your mind continuing to whirl for a much longer period of time before actually getting to sleep. The best way to fall asleep is via an indirect route of relaxing your mind and letting go of thoughts about sleep.

If it takes you 5 minutes or less to fall asleep, you may not be getting enough total sleep or quality sleep. Although your SE could be very high (and who doesn't like seeing a score of 98% on a report?) this could be a good indicator that you should seek out a more comprehensive physiological evaluation regarding your sleep.

SLEEP LOG

Date	6/12/16		
Bed Time (BT) What time did you get into bed?	11:15 pm		
Lights Out (LO) What time did you try to go to sleep?	12:45 am		
Sleep Onset Latency (SOL) How long did it take you to fall asleep?	55 min		
How many times did you wake up?	2 times		
Wake After Sleep Onset (WASO) How long was each of your awakenings?	1 Hour 15 min		
Wake Time (WT) What time was your final awakening?	6:35 am		
Rise Time (RT) What time did you get out of bed?	7:45 am		
Time in Bed (TIB)	8.5 hours		
Total Sleep Time (TST)	3.75 hours		

EXERCISE: INTERPRETING YOUR
SLEEP PATTERNS

After you complete the first week of your sleep log, you'll
start to uncover meaningful information about your sleep
patterns. At this point you'll be able to start identifying
which parts of your sleep are healthy and which parts could
use a tune-up. Here are some questions to start you off:

1. What was it like to track your sleep for this past week?

_____

_____

2. Did any patterns immediately jump out at you?

_____

_____

3. Did any patterns surprise you?

_____

_____

4. What are you already doing well?

_____

_____

5. Is there anything you may want to change?

_____

_____

IDENTIFYING UNHEALTHY SLEEP

As you continue to examine your sleep patterns, see if you identify with any of these prevalent signs of unhealthy sleep. In Chapter 2, unhealthy sleep is defined as suboptimal-quantity or low-quality sleep. It can manifest in several different forms, from an outlier event such as an all-nighter to a more chronic condition such as a sleep disorder. Below are a few scenarios to help you identify where you may fall in the spectrum of unhealthy sleep.

Falling Asleep Too Quickly

There is a common misperception that falling asleep quickly is a sign of a "good sleeper." But if you find yourself falling asleep as soon as your head touches the pillow, or even outside of the bedroom, it may indicate excessive sleepiness. These could be signs of chronic sleep deprivation and potentially sleep apnea.

When you are properly rested, it should normally take anywhere from 10 to 20 minutes to fall asleep. Your body is not a machine you can just switch off, so winding it down takes a few minutes. Evolutionarily, sleep was quite a dangerous activity because it left our ancestors unable to defend themselves from predators or rivals. Making sure that the environment was safe for the duration of our slumber would have been critical for survival, so developing a gradual transition period likely allowed us to safely drift to sleep while still listening for danger.

Falling Asleep Too Slowly

When you begin spending more than 30 minutes trying to fall asleep, that's when your efforts become counterproductive. This can lead to watching the clock, tossing in bed, and frustration that you're not asleep already. The majority of people will experience this for at least one night over the course of their lifetime, if not several nights. Growing anticipation on the eve of receiving holiday gifts, a major exam, a new job, or an exciting trip can leave one lying awake imagining what the future will reveal. Life is full of these events and, fortunately, they usually cause only minor blips on one's sleep radar.

Trouble starts brewing when you find yourself regularly stringing together several of these sleepless nights in a row. The more we lie awake in bed, the more our bodies are conditioned to remain awake and not asleep in bed. This can easily lead to chronic sleep loss and could be a sign of insomnia.

Waking Up Frequently

Are you waking up too many times at night? Or spending too much time awake at night? We naturally drift in and out of periods of light sleep throughout the night as we cycle through our sleep rhythms. Even though we are more susceptible to being awoken, we normally continue to sleep through until the morning. As we age, we have a greater propensity to wake up during these periods at night but usually are able to return to sleep within a few minutes.

One or two awakenings of this variety are probably not disruptive enough to be an issue unless they keep you awake for longer than 30 minutes. Similar to difficulties falling asleep, spending significant amounts of time awake at night may condition your body to associate the bed with wakefulness.

If the frequency increases beyond three awakenings per night consistently, it is worth noting. Even if it is only for a few minutes each time, the cumulative effect of these disruptions can begin eating away at your total nightly sleep. For example, if you begin to notice that you are waking up several times a night, it could be useful to pay attention to the potential causes. If you get up because you need to use the restroom, you may be drinking liquids too close to bedtime. If frequent nighttime bathroom visits persist even after you reduce your liquid intake at night, you may want to seek further medical evaluation because it could be a sign of a sleep disorder (e.g., sleep apnea, nightmares, night terrors, restless leg syndrome) or another physiological issue. Frequent nighttime awakenings can also be caused by environmental factors such as ambient noise, temperature, light, pets, or your bed partner, so carefully evaluating how much these influence your sleep can help you take appropriate steps to minimize their impact.

Snoring

"It's perfectly normal to snore" is a common myth associated with being a "good sleeper"; the truth is quite the opposite. Snoring is caused by a partial or complete blockage of the airway, which is as bad as it sounds. This blockage equates to reduced oxygen levels to the brain and body; without enough oxygen our brain cells will begin to die. Snoring is also associated with obstructive sleep apnea. The long-term effects of sleep apnea include weight gain, hypertension, cardiovascular disease, diabetes, memory loss, and in extreme cases death. The presence of snoring does not always indicate sleep apnea but is worth evaluating if you notice it happening. As I shared in the introduction to this book, I was one of these folks and can definitely relate to the chronic sleepiness caused by this disorder.

Grinding Teeth

Do you clench or grind your teeth at night? Do you wake up with jaw pain and morning headaches? Another noisy nighttime companion that may indicate sleep apnea is teeth grinding, or bruxism. If you've ever heard someone grinding his or her teeth while sleeping, it can be a grating experience. Often someone who has bruxism doesn't realize they suffer from it until a visit to the dentist or a sleep partner mentions it.

The link between your dental health and sleep is an ingenious safety mechanism of the body. If your brain recognizes that your breathing is being restricted while you sleep, it will switch on just enough power to activate your jaw muscles. This clenching tightens the tissue around your airway and allows for air to travel unimpeded. The downside, aside from needing dentures several years before retirement, is that flicking on extraneous brain processes at night can also kick you out of your deep sleep and bounce you around in lighter stages. So if either of these "sound sleeping" warning signs, snoring or teeth grinding, are happening to you regularly, it could be time to get it professionally evaluated.

Falling Asleep During the Day

Do you notice yourself falling asleep at inappropriate times during the day? That classic slow dip of the head followed by a sudden jerk of the body back to wakefulness and wide eyes when you're in class, in a meeting, or even on the drive home? This is called a micro sleep and is also a sign that you may need more or better quality sleep. Even moderate sleep loss (1 to 2 hours below your optimal sleep duration for a few nights) can increase the presence of micro sleeps when the sleep loss becomes chronic.

Another sign of daytime sleepiness is called sleep attacks. This typically happens when someone begins a physically passive activity such as sitting in a meeting. A sleep-starved body will jump at this opportunity of inactivity and suddenly initiate the onset of sleep. It can be a frustrating experience because some people remain conscious enough to try to fight the sleep attack but are powerless to stop it. And unlike a micro sleep, a sleep attack can last much longer depending on how much sleep debt the individual has accrued and could be a sign of narcolepsy. So if you are experiencing any of these for extended periods of time, particularly sleep attacks, it could be a good time to connect with a sleep specialist.

Sleeping in on Weekends

Sleeping in on weekends is one of the most common indicators of sleep debt. It is often tempting after a long, challenging week to sleep in on the weekend. It feels great to let go of outside pressures and can be a delicious treat after a hard week. Unfortunately, sleeping in throws a significant wrench into the gears of your sleep clock by knocking your sleep homeostat out of sync with your circadian rhythm. When you wake up 3 hours later than you do on workdays, your sleep drive has 3 fewer hours to build by bedtime. So even though your circadian clock will release melatonin after dusk to get the rest of your body ready for sleep, you will be unable to fall asleep at your normal bedtime because you just won't feel sleepy enough.

This dyssynchrony between your biological clock and external clock happens in a similar fashion when traveling across time zones and is commonly referred to as jet lag. Your cellular clocks can't reset at the same speed as a plane, which leaves you trying to fit your East Coast rhythms into a West Coast lifestyle. Appetite, alertness, and even physical performance lag behind and can take up to 24 hours to resynchronize for each time zone crossed. Anticipating these changes leading up to a trip, combined with a few behavioral adjustments, can help you accelerate your adjustment before you get to your next destination. Calculating the precise combination of appropriately timed dim light, bright light, low doses of melatonin, and shifted bed and wake times to help you adapt more quickly goes beyond the scope of this book. Fortunately, there are several free apps and websites that can help you calculate a jet lag sleep schedule.

When to Seek Professional Help

Everyone has a different threshold for making an appointment to see a health professional. Some people may go in at the slightest inkling of concern, while others may hold out until other people drag them there. With regard to sleep health, most people tend to lean toward the latter because there is little public awareness of the short- and long-term risks of poor sleep health. It is often viewed as nonessential to functioning and not worth the cost of making a visit to the local clinic.

If you resonated with a few of the above scenarios, my professional recommendation is to talk to your physician about it sooner rather than later. This can be helpful in improving your quality of life and preventing more serious health issues later on.

Also, it's important to note that our daytime fatigue may be related to other mental and physical health conditions such as depression, anxiety, trauma, chronic pain, thyroid issues, or infections. It can be easy to blame sleep or the lack thereof for our fatigue and sleepiness. Remembering that there are numerous other factors that may contribute to feeling worn down can help us determine if there are other facets of life that could improve our energy with the proper attention.

PUTTING IT ALL TOGETHER

The sleep log is a quick way to start gathering data points about our sleeping patterns. Though it can be a lot of technical information to digest, starting with one day can help you get the sleep train rolling.

For people who prefer to engage on a more narrative and descriptive level, the next chapter on your sleep story may be a more natural place to begin. Understanding our thought patterns, emotions, and behaviors provides a fantastic complement to our quantitative sleep data and an even richer picture of our sleep.

Chapter 4

SLEEP STORY

As you begin to build awareness around your sleep patterns, you'll start to notice that certain thoughts and emotions are informing your behaviors around sleeping. This steady dialogue has developed over time and influences why you do things a certain way. I like to call these our sleep stories.

When we're sleep deprived, we think about needing more sleep but often rationalize why we can't get enough through a specific story that reflects our present reality: *I just started a new job and there's a steep learning curve, so I have to work overtime to understand my role. I have a new puppy and need to make sure it is happy and doesn't pee on my carpet when I'm not looking. I recently moved across the country and am adjusting to new surroundings, new friends, and a new time zone.* Any of these sound familiar? We have all been there at some point in our lives. These narratives can reassure us that our sleep loss is temporary and that we will eventually return to our normal sleep routines when the stressors fade away.

However, if we carry these kinds of stories beyond their usefulness, they can continue to influence our sleep even after the temporary stressors have subsided. To tease apart the elements of our stories that continue to be helpful from ones that are no longer useful, you can categorize them into three buckets: thoughts, emotions, and behaviors that affect your sleep. As you start to take the time to tune into your various stories, you will begin to see how each facet can influence the others and in turn help or hinder your sleep.

EXERCISE: WHAT'S MY SLEEP STORY?

Let's start by asking these questions:

1. What is my relationship with sleep? Draw the image that comes to mind.

2. What am I telling myself about how well I sleep?

_____

_____

_____

3. What am I feeling about my sleep quality?

_____

_____

_____

4. What am I doing about my sleep health?

_____

_____

_____

These prompts can help draw out the components of your sleep story and illuminate the connections between your thoughts, emotions, and behaviors. In the introduction, I shared with you my own initial story: *I sleep so well that I can*

sleep through an earthquake; I must be one of the lucky ones.
The image that I drew was of me happily snoring through the
night with a big smile on my face. In my mind, I was a good
sleeper (thought), who felt fortunate to have a positive relationship with going to bed (emotion), and I treated myself by
sleeping in on the weekend (behavior). By starting here, I was
able to notice what I was telling myself.

If we can build our awareness around the connections
between our minds and our actions, then we can start recognizing what may be contributing to a particular bout of
sleep disruption and do something about it.

THOUGHTS

Why are our thoughts so important? They serve as the basis
for how we think about ourselves, relate to others, and how
we find meaning in this world. In this chapter, we'll discuss
them in the context of how they influence our emotions and
our behaviors.

According to the Laboratory of Neuroimaging at the University of Southern California, adults average 70,000 thoughts
per waking day. That's about one thought per second! So it's
no surprise that when we are about to fall asleep, a cascade
of enticing and numerous musings, which have been held at
bay all day, come pouring in. It can be incredibly tempting to
grab hold of at least one or two of them and see where they
take us. Some can be highly engaging, like replaying scenes
from an exciting movie you just watched, or others can be

anxiety provoking like scanning through your growing to-do list for tomorrow. Others may begin more innocuously, such as the sound of a car alarm outside triggering thoughts of wondering if you locked your car or not, or thinking about a task you have to complete at work tomorrow. Those can lead to another action item that you have to do the following day, or remind you of a conversation you had with an inspiring coworker the week prior.

Within a few seconds of unconsciously grasping onto a single thought, a flood of memories, ideas, and associations ripple out, keeping our minds churning and our bodies awake. Any thought can make it more difficult for us to really let go of the day and fall asleep. For many people, one thought can get replayed over and over again and impact them for a few nights or even weeks at a time. When the challenges of falling asleep become more consistent, *thoughts* of trying to fall asleep can also start entering the mind, feeding the active brain instead of shutting it down. These myriad associations can eventually begin to link thinking with bedtime and contribute to difficulties falling asleep even when exhausted.

The wise approach is to choose which thoughts you want to continue to follow and which ones to release. Becoming more aware of your thoughts, especially as bedtime approaches, can help you recognize unhelpful thinking patterns that interfere with your sleep. This awareness can help you avert potential sleeplessness. The intentional practice of recognizing and acknowledging a constant stream of thoughts will give you the option of continuing to follow them or not.

EXERCISE: LEAVES ON A STREAM

This guided meditation is a great tool to help you begin to train yourself to become more aware of your thoughts without getting swept up in them.

- Find a comfortable position, either seated or lying down. Close your eyes, and start by taking a few full, deep breaths, all the way in, and all the way out.

- When you're ready, allow your breath to return to its normal pace and rhythm, and notice the quality of it. Is the exhalation longer than the inhalation? Is there a brief pause at the top or the bottom? Is your breathing effortful or effortless? At this point there is no need to change it; simply notice the slow and relaxed inhale followed by an easy and relaxed exhale.

- As you sit with your breath, imagine you are sitting on the bank of a stream. You feel the warmth of the sun directly overhead and as you look out onto the stream, you notice several large, colorful leaves drifting slowly along in the current. As you observe the stream, take a few moments to notice what you see, hear, smell, and feel.

- When you're ready, begin to notice your thoughts. They may be plans for the future, memories of the past, or judgments of self or others. Whatever they are, try to observe them for simply what they are without hooking onto any one thought.

- As the thoughts come into your awareness, imagine placing each on its own leaf one by one, and watch as the leaves gently carry the thoughts out of view.

- Some leaves may bounce along the currents and swiftly carry thoughts away, while others may get caught in small eddies and swirl around for a few moments before slowly drifting downstream. Or, perhaps, a leaf may carry one thought away, just to have that same thought reappear. Whatever the case, if you find yourself focusing on recurrent thoughts or ones that continue to hang around, simply acknowledge that it is happening and gently return your attention to the arising of thoughts, placing each one on a leaf, and watching it float away.

- After spending a few minutes noticing the thoughts come and go, allow the thoughts and image of the stream to slowly fade and return your attention to your breath. Notice the quality of it. Is your exhalation longer than the inhalation? Is there a brief pause at the top and the bottom? Is it effortful or effortless? Begin to notice more sounds in the room, feel sensation return to your body and extremities, and slowly open your eyes when you're ready.

1. What was that experience like for you?

_____

_____

2. What did you notice?

_____

_____

_____

_____

It takes time to become adept at noticing our thoughts. Even people who have meditated for years can find themselves far away from the present moment lost in rumination. However, each time we practice disengaging from a distracting thought, we continue to groove those neuropathways of noticing our thoughts and making the choice to let them go. This small act of conscious, intentional living returns us to our present experience. Subsequently, we feel more relaxed and at ease because we can more fully enjoy what we are doing instead of worrying about what we did or what we should do in the future.

EMOTIONS

Sleep can be an emotional experience; it can evoke the entire range of feelings from bliss to anxiety to terror. Building up your reservoir of positive emotional associations with sleep will help strengthen your motivation to resume your sleep practice when it gets out of tune.

Those whose sleep experiences evoke negative emotional associations can have an aversion to nighttime and sleep. Some people may consider sleeping a waste of time and build an unconscious resentment toward it. Others who have experienced significant trauma may have recurrent nightmares that recall traumatic events and subsequently develop a fear of falling asleep. Having such negative emotional connections can build strong barriers against the entire process. The more irritated and frustrated you become while trying to sleep, the more activated your body and mind becomes, feeding your restlessness. Identifying negative emotional associations that impact your sleep can give you additional insights into triggers that disrupt your sleep and how to mitigate them before they become problematic.

As powerful drivers of our experiences, how can we become more intentional in harnessing our emotions? One of the approaches is to notice how your emotion shows up in your body, or somatically. Our perceptions of a thought, a smell, or a situation can trigger a chain reaction of physiological responses and associated memories. An emotion, or feeling, is often identified by the sensations it generates in our minds and bodies. Anxiety, for example, is commonly experienced in the head and body as reddened cheeks, flushed ears, racing thoughts, shallow breathing, and tightness in the chest. The feeling of dread, on the other hand, is often felt in the pit of the stomach. Building awareness of the physiological manifestations of our emotions can be important clues into our moment-to-moment experience.

EXERCISE: TUNING IN TO YOUR EMOTIONS

Just as with your thoughts, setting aside time to intentionally pay attention to your emotions will help you become more consistently attuned to them as they are happening. The following exercise can help you notice the different sensations your body may produce with contrasting emotions.

- Find a comfortable position, either seated or lying down. Close your eyes, and start by taking a few full, deep breaths, all the way in, and all the way out.

- When you're ready, allow your breath to return to its normal pace and rhythm, and notice the quality of it. Is the exhalation longer than the inhalation? Is there a brief pause at the top or the bottom? Is it effortful or effortless?

- At this point there is no need to change it; simply notice the slow and relaxed inhale followed by an easy and relaxed exhale.

- As you sit here with your breath, now imagine a recent situation where you had troubling falling asleep. It could be following a heated argument with a loved one, continuing to solve a challenging problem at work, or coming back from an overseas trip and your days and nights are all jumbled up. When the specific memory comes to mind, notice the different thoughts, feelings, and sensations that arise. Thoughts of where you were and feelings of frustration or anger may bubble to the surface.

- As they do, notice any sensations in your body as well. You may feel tightness in your shoulders or chest; your heart rate may quicken; or you may feel flushed and warm. As you draw your attention to your emotions and sensations, see if you can observe them as they are and without judgment. Notice how your body and mind react to these emotions as you continue to sit in the experience.

- On your next exhalation, blow out that experience. Take another deep inhalation and allow the thoughts, emotions, and sensations of that memory to fade as you exhale slowly.

- As your breath returns to its normal pace and rhythm, now bring to mind the memory of a time when you slept well. When the specific memory comes to mind, notice the different thoughts, feelings, and sensations that arise. Thoughts of where you were and feelings of perhaps peacefulness or happiness may bubble to the surface.

- As they do, notice any sensations in your body as well. This time you may feel relaxation or lightness in your shoulders; your heart rate may quicken or slow; or you may find yourself smiling. As you draw your attention to your emotions and sensations, see if you can observe them as they are, again without judgment. Notice how your body and mind react to these emotions as you continue to sit in the experience.

- Finally, on your next exhalation, blow out that experience. Take another deep inhalation and allow the thoughts, emotions, and sensations of that memory to fade as you exhale slowly. As your breath returns to its normal pace and rhythm, once again note the quality of it. Begin to notice more sounds in the room, feel sensation return to your body and extremities, and slowly open your eyes when you're ready.

1. How was that experience for you?

_____

_____

2. What came up for you?

_____

_____

3. Did you notice any changes in your breath or body when you went between the two memories?

_____

_____

As you continue to heighten your sensitivity to your emotions and the physiological responses they elicit in your body, you can acknowledge them and choose whether you want to intensify them or allow them to gently pass. Just like with your thoughts, each time you recognize an emotion and decide to continue following it or to let it go the likelihood that you will be able to recognize it again increases. With practice, you will become aware of these sensations closer to the triggering event and be able to make that choice earlier. The sooner you can recognize an emotion that may impede your sleep, the more effectively you will be able to employ this practice as part of your early warning system for sleeplessness.

BEHAVIORS

Behaviors can be defined as an observable response to an internal or external stimuli. What we do is often influenced by what we are thinking and feeling. Whether it's unconscious or not, it's what those around us see, hear, and feel. So what we do around our sleep and wake routines can provide a great opportunity to identify unhealthy habits that are reducing the quality of our sleep.

For example, one of the most common activities that affects our sleep is using digital devices the hour before we fall asleep. This includes phones, tablets, computers, and televisions. Why? Because the screens emit bright or blue-wave light that, keeps us alert. Our bodies will only begin to release melatonin, the hormone that makes us sleepy, once we stop exposing our eyes to bright lights. Even with the new light dimming filters, such as f.lux or Apple's Night Shift, research has shown that continuing to use our devices right up until bedtime can still disrupt our sleep if the content of the media is too engaging. Now let's say part of your sleep story is "scrolling through my Facebook feed helps me fall asleep." You may be thinking "this is a good way to decompress," but what's actually happening is that your screen time may be delaying the release of melatonin or activating your brain, causing you to take more time to fall asleep. So it's important to take a look at all the behaviors surrounding your sleep to see which ones are helping or hindering.

EXERCISE: WHAT BEHAVIORS IMPACT MY SLEEP?

List what activities you do before falling asleep and after waking up. After completing your list, follow the directions on page 104.

Bed Time - What I do before falling asleep:

Wake Time - What I do after waking up:

Bed Time:

Circle items that may be activating (exercising, sending emails, reading an exciting novel, scrolling through social media, etc).

- Place a "−" next to the activities with bright lights or screens

- Place a "Δ" next to the activities you are doing in bed

- Place a "+" next to activities that are non-work, don't involve screen time, outside your bedroom, or relaxing

Wake Time:

- Place a Δ if you are using the snooze button or lying in bed for longer than 30 minutes

- Place a + next to activities that help you start your day (meditating, exercising, eating breakfast, getting exposure to bright light, etc.)

- Any interesting patterns?

IMPACT

Now that you have a better sense of your sleep story, let's take it to the next level by exploring how it affects not only you, but also those around you.

EXERCISE: WHAT IS THE IMPACT OF MY SLEEP?

How does my sleep impact me?

How does my sleep impact my sleep?

Is there anything I want to change about my sleep?

1. Any interesting patterns?

_____

_____

_____

_____

2. Any insights or surprises?

_____

_____

_____

_____

If you're finding yourself coming to some quick conclusions or resistance, consider shifting your approach to one that starts with curiosity and without judgment. For me, it was moving from "I've always slept in on weekends so there's no need to change that now" to "How interesting that I've always slept in. I wonder why that is?" In mindfulness, this attitude is called *beginner's mind,* in which you try to approach situations, even seemingly mundane or routine ones, as novel and

worthy of your full attention. In relation to sleep, this attitude allows us to remove preconceived ideas we may hold
that can limit our perspective and evaluate our current sleep
habits with fresh eyes.

PUTTING IT ALL TOGETHER

By this point, you've undertaken a meaningful effort to assess
your habits, patterns, and perspectives through the sleep log
and sleep story exercises. Hopefully, you're starting to see
how the activities you engage in around bed and wake time
can affect your sleep.

Through building this awareness, you can more effectively
recognize and then intentionally choose the approach you
want to take. In the next section, we will focus on strategies
around your sleep environment.

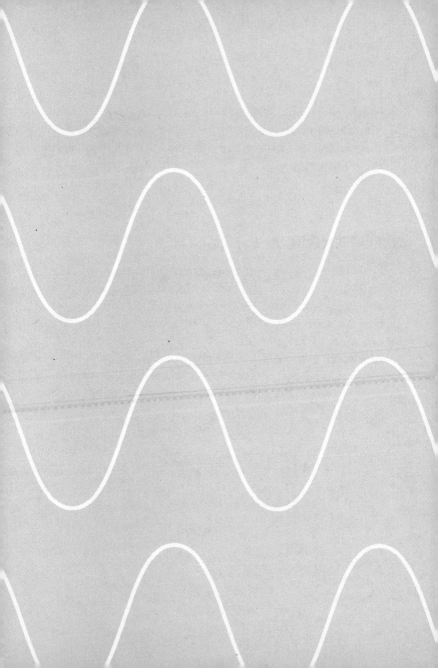

Chapter 5

SLEEP ENVIRONMENT

Cultivating a comfortable and relaxing environment is a great first step toward improving our sleep. It's relatively easy to implement, can be fun to do, and is an opportune excuse to form healthy routines. Our sleep environment is part of the broader set of practices we call *sleep hygiene,* or habits conducive to sleeping well and feeling awake. The primary purpose is to reinforce positive associations with sleep. Whether it's the comfort of our beds or the space to decompress, creating as many pleasant connections as possible will make sleep more enjoyable so that we look forward to it. Establishing these connections appropriately at the beginning will facilitate the ease with which we can sustain positive changes to our sleep.

If you've been collecting data for your sleep log, this is the ideal time to focus on your sleep environment. We are often so tempted to jump right in and fix our sleep schedules that we run past our surroundings. Tactically, it actually takes a couple of weeks to get a more accurate picture of our typical sleep patterns. I usually recommended my clients complete their sleep log for two weeks before adjusting their sleep patterns. So while you're collecting, let's start making a sleep-friendly space.

In this chapter we will discuss strategies for optimizing our beds and bedrooms for a high-quality night of rest. Keep in mind that what is comfortable and relaxing is somewhat different for each of us. So experiment with what works for you by noticing what calms you down versus what makes you restless.

YOUR BED

It seems matter-of-fact that our beds are for sleeping. However, as more people are working from home, many of us are regularly using our beds for other activities such as writing emails and watching shows. As the lines blur, we get used to being active and awake in bed.

What we end up doing is conditioning our bodies and minds to associate being awake with being in bed. This process is based on the work of Russian physiologist Ivan Pavlov, who popularized Pavlovian response after his famous study with his dogs. During one of his experiments, while examining the saliva output in response to dog food powder, he inadvertently discovered that his dogs would begin salivating when he entered the room even before presenting them with the dog food. He quickly ascertained that the dogs had reflexively "learned" to associate his presence with food, which caused them to salivate even in the absence of food. This process, known as *classical conditioning,* is incredibly adaptive because it allows animals and humans to unconsciously anticipate likely outcomes from their environment. Using this principle of establishing automatic associations will allow you to train your body to unconsciously anticipate sleep when you get into bed.

For Sleep & Sex, Not Texts

Our beds are for sleep and sex *only.* If you skip reading this entire chapter, and implement only this discipline, I'd consider my work here a success. It may sound simple or even trivial, but developing this association will train your body and mind to keep thoughts, worries, and work outside of the bedroom and unconnected with sleep. This idea, called *stimulus control,* permeates many of the sleep strategies we will discuss and has also been shown to help shift sleep as a standalone intervention.

By carefully and intentionally limiting the number of activities we do in bed, our bodies and minds will begin to disassociate dynamic activities with our beds. For example, if you take a nap during the day, use your bed instead of the couch. This will strengthen the sleep-bed connection and weaken any associations between sleep and other environments. Separating these states is critical to both weakening the associations between wakefulness and our

beds while strengthening the bond between sleeping and
our beds. This is particularly important during bouts of
insomnia or when our sleep is knocked out of alignment.

Keep Work Out

Every client that I have worked with has taken work to
bed multiple nights per week whether it be studying, work
emails, reports, or presentations. Limiting the amount of
work we do in the bedroom as much as possible, and stop-
ping it as early in the day as possible, can also help weaken
the association between sleep and our thinking minds.

For most of my life, I was no different and brazenly kept
my desk in my bedroom with negligible consequences. In
my 500-square-foot one-bedroom apartment there weren't
many options. It wasn't until I began writing my disser-
tation that I noticed my mind was racing in bed; it could
no longer make the distinction between thinking time at
my desk and thinking time in my bed. Applying stimulus
control, I moved my desk just outside my bedroom door.
Within a week, my mind and body were able to quickly
compartmentalize "thinking" to outside of my bedroom. I
was falling asleep with ease. By moving the desk even just
a few feet away, my mind was able to keep sleep and relaxation on one side of the door and reading, intellectualizing,
and writing on the other side.

I was fortunate enough to have the space to separate the
two, but for many people this may not be feasible. One of
the common realities of living with one or more beings, be
they family, friends, or pets, is a limitation on space, which

can push the desk back into the bedroom. In those cases, it is critical that the bed itself is reserved for sleep and sex. If you are unable to work or study in other areas of your home and find your sleep disrupted by these activities occurring in your bedroom, it may be time to find an external location. A nearby coffee house or local library are great places to let your creative and working mind range free to help keep your bedroom just for sleep and sex.

Lounge Elsewhere

Limit your lounging, reading, and media in bed. For some of us lounging in bed is helpful for falling asleep. These leisure activities, while relaxing, can be detrimental to our sleep in a couple of ways. They can either be too engaging, watching a hilarious show that unintentionally keeps us awake past our desired bedtime, or too relaxing, reading reports that accidentally put us to sleep too early in the day. Even with automatic timers, the flicker from the TV or lamp can disrupt our stages of sleep. In either case, it is wise to start getting into the habit of shifting those activities to other environments for the benefit of your sleep.

Make Your Bed

Our parents had it right all along! Making our beds when we get up gives us a sense of accomplishment, creates a positive mood, and leads to a cleaner bedroom. Smoothing out the comforter and resetting your pillow only takes a few seconds and will keep your bed clean and tidy for when you return in the evening.

Making our beds also helps us reduce the desire to get back into bed for additional sleep. The grogginess we often feel when we wake up, known as sleep inertia, can make falling back asleep seem like a great idea. That is perfectly normal even when we are properly rested. Going back to sleep at this point is counterproductive because it gets us accustomed to fragmenting our sleep. Getting up immediately and making your bed will place a small but significant barrier to getting back into bed until your sleep inertia wears off and you feel energized to continue your day.

Make It Comfortable

Lastly, our beds are personal spaces. It is often one of the few places that is relaxing and safe; a sanctuary where we can retreat from the outside world every day. So making it as comfortable as possible is in our best interest. With my clients, I may ask if their mattress is the correct level of firmness. One that is too soft or too hard can leave us feeling sore and unrested in the morning. The comfort of their linens can also be an important part of this discussion. Our bedding should be breathable, provide us enough warmth, and be comfortable to the touch. Correlational research linked fresh, or fresh-smelling bedding, with greater relaxation when getting into bed, so even the smell of your sheets may have a small impact on your sleep. Perhaps this is a good excuse to swap out that old mattress and comforter for a new one?

YOUR BEDROOM

Our surroundings play an important role in allowing our senses to relax to the point where we can let go and fall asleep. Ensuring that our bedrooms are comfortable and conducive to sleep is also intuitive, but it's important to reiterate because we have tendencies to let unhealthy habits creep into the bedroom.

Leave Devices Out

Following "bed is for sleep and sex," a device-free bed and bedroom is the next most important element. But as electronic devices have become so multifunctional, removing them from our bedrooms can take some getting used to. As we know from the science of sleep, artificial light, particularly from sources that emit blue-wave light such as TVs, computer screens, and smartphones, is disruptive and may delay the release of melatonin. But most of us have come to form strong attachments to our devices; they provide us connectedness, security, and entertainment. So creating and adhering to boundaries regarding these devices can be very challenging. And they are definitely achievable.

For my clients, I recommend a two-pronged strategy: temporal distance and physical distance. *Temporal distance* refers to slowly increasing the time between last screen use and bedtime, ideally 60–90 minutes before bed. Start with 5 minutes, and then gradually increase in 10-minute increments until you reach your optimal time. *Physical distance* pushes the devices away from the bed, ideally outside the bedroom. Start with moving your devices off your bed onto your nightstand, eventually leaving it in another part of your home. This is critical for placing a physical barrier to responding immediately. The buzz and pings from our phone actually stimulate a dopamine hit, causing our brains to become addicted to seek texts, email, and social media feeds. We can turn off the dopamine loop by putting our phones on the "Do Not Disturb" mode, silencing the notifications, or placing the phone with the screen facing down. If your phone doubles as an alarm clock, consider getting a stand-alone or an analog one.

Keep It Dark

Now that our bedrooms are delightfully device-free, we can focus on reducing the external light coming into the room. Ever notice how most hotel rooms have blackout curtains? Light is the most powerful cue our body uses to differentiate when to sleep and when to be active. Keeping a dark room, absent of blinking devices and night-lights, will provide unambiguous signals that it is time for sleep.

During summer months, when the sun sets later and rises earlier, it can be easy get be thrown off our sleep schedules because the amount of natural darkness shrinks. If you have windows in your bedroom that receive morning sunlight or artificial light from street lamps, getting blackout curtains is a popular method for managing the darkness in your bedroom.

Keep It Cool

As mentioned earlier, our bodies naturally experience a drop in core temperature when we fall asleep. While the exact mechanism is still being researched, a lower body temperature may help regulate the circadian rhythms of certain organs and lower our metabolism to conserve energy at night. Maintaining a room that is slightly cooler will facilitate this process.

The National Sleep Foundation recommends ambient temperatures between 65 to 72 degrees Fahrenheit. Some people may fall outside of this range, so finding the ideal temperature for you may take a little tinkering. If you are unsure of your bedroom's temperature, just make sure that it is cooler than the room you were in prior to going to bed. There is some research that suggests that mimicking our body's temperature drop as we drift to sleep may be just as important as a cool ambient temperature. Whatever temperature you select, just remember to make it comfortable for you: when our bedrooms are too cold or too hot, the discomfort can delay or interrupt our sleep.

Keep It Quiet

In general, having a quiet room for sleep allows for the most peaceful sleep. Minimal noise allows us to relax and fall asleep quicker and stay asleep. However, sound is a little more nuanced than darkness because we generally sleep best in environments where the sounds, or lack thereof, are familiar. For example, people who live in cities often describe difficulties sleeping in the countryside because it is too quiet. Paradoxically, their brains have gotten so used to the constant noise of the city that the complete absence of noise puts the brain on alert because it is so unusual.

If you identify with being more sensitive to sound, you may benefit from earplugs or adding a constant sound to your sleep environment, such as a white noise machine. Your brain will soon adjust to it and will quickly begin to associate that noise with sleep. This will also allow you to bring this cue along with you when you travel which can help your body feel more at ease when you're away from your home.

Keep It Clean

Keeping our bedrooms clean keeps our minds peaceful when we enter, and makes it more relaxing to stay. A few studies have shown that having cluttered, messy sleeping spaces can contribute to difficulties sleeping; the messiness can begin to regularly stimulate and irritate, rather than relax, our minds when we enter our bedroom. Clutter for many people can trigger thoughts of never-ending household chores: fold the laundry, sort the mail, file the papers, organize the closet, and the list goes on. These thoughts often float in the background, but can steadily drain our energy and add to the bucket of sleep disruptions.

For some, maintaining a clean room comes naturally, but for others, it can take some strategizing. As you assess your bedroom, notice what types of clutter tends to accumulate in your space. Where do clothes, books, and accessories gather? Where do you put down your bag? Where do you leave your work clothes? Some people try on several outfits before heading out and leave the unused pieces on the floor or bed. This can quickly add up to several discarded outfits strewn across the room after only a couple of days. Replacing clothes you don't use after making your decision will help maintain your room. Implementing a few practices can help with this maintenance. I find that it is easier to maintain a clean room rather than clean up a messy one. If you continue to feel rushed in the mornings, reduce your anxiety by picking out your clothes the night before. It sounds basic, but it is something that I frequently suggest to my clients because it is effective.

PUTTING IT ALL TOGETHER

Much of what we covered here is no surprise; they are everyday elements of mindful living. Taken together, these timeless rituals help us establish a sleep environment that enables us to have a pleasant relationship with sleep. Sometimes we just need a nudge to get us back in our flow.

....

EXERCISE: HOW MINDFUL IS MY SLEEP ENVIRONMENT?

....

Circle the answers that best describe your sleep environment on a typical night.

MY BED

Do I use my bed just for sleep and sex?	Yes	Sometimes	No
Do I leave my work out of my bed?	Yes	Sometimes	No
Do I leave devices out of my bed?	Yes	Sometimes	No
Do I lounge outside of my bed?	Yes	Sometimes	No
Is my bedding comfortable?	Yes	Sometimes	No
Is my mattress comfortable?	Yes	Sometimes	No
Do I make my bed?	Yes	Sometimes	No

MY BEDROOM

Do I leave my devices out of the bedroom?	Yes	Sometimes	No
Do I silence my devices when I sleep?	Yes	Sometimes	No
Do I work outside of my bedroom?	Yes	Sometimes	No
Is the temperature cool enough to fall asleep?	Yes	Sometimes	No
Is my bedroom quiet enough to fall asleep?	Yes	Sometimes	No
Is my room dark and free of bright light?	Yes	Sometimes	No
Is my bedroom clean and free of clutter?	Yes	Sometimes	No

1. Circle the three environmental factors that have the most detrimental impact on your sleep.

2. Make a star by the three that are the easiest for you to address.

3. Any patterns, insights, or surprises?

_____

_____

_____

_____

Undeniably, as the business of life accelerates, even our sanctuary can get neglected, so it is helpful to periodically reevaluate. If you can make your room comfortable, cool, quiet, and dark, you're on your way to making a sleep-friendly space. Making adjustments to all arenas at once can be daunting. If it feels overwhelming to implement all of these changes at once, pick one that feels the most doable and slowly incorporate the rest of the suggestions at your own pace.

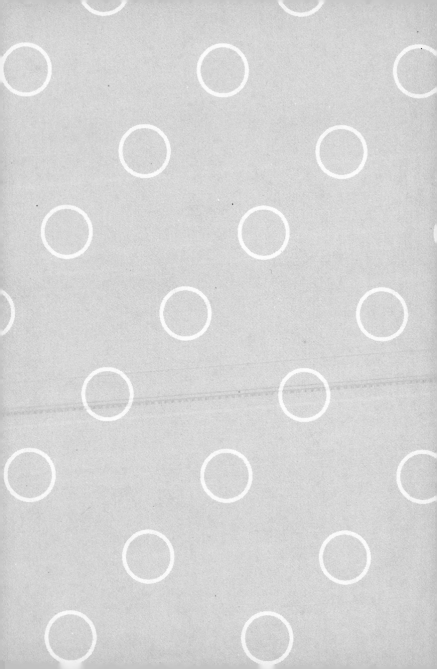

Chapter 6

SLEEP SCHEDULE

Our sleep, like any skill, can be mastered through consistent, intentional practice; the more deliberate our effort, the more beneficial it is for our health. By tracking your sleep and improving your sleep environment, you are beginning to practice healthy sleep habits. It's important for us to acknowledge these meaningful first steps because we don't necessarily "see" the changes during this seeding period. And we can easily digress to "It's not working, forget it." What we're doing is laying the mental groundwork, signaling to our brains that we're ingraining new patterns of behavior. Contrary to popular belief, motivation *follows* action; each incremental step gives us the boost of motivation to continue. And as we enter this next stage, the new neural pathways we've built will be key to our sleep success.

We're now ready to enter the core of behavioral sleep medicine: *sleep scheduling*. This is where we work to build a consistent sleep schedule, over a period of 8 weeks, to improve both our quality and quantity of sleep. In shifting away from poor sleep habits to optimal sleep strategies week by week, we begin to see the most notable changes in how we feel.

Intuitive in nature, sleep scheduling forms the basis for cognitive behavioral therapy for insomnia. This treatment is widely studied and empirically validated; up to 80% of clients who complete the program will have very few or no symptoms at the end of treatment. Its benefits are generally seen to be equally or more effective than medication in the short-term and superior in the long-term. As with any behavioral change, these strategies will not improve your sleep overnight; it will take persistence and patience to realize the benefits.

Baseline data from your sleep log is necessary to effectively move forward. So, if you haven't started the sleep log exercise from Chapter 3, I would recommend doing that now.

LEARN YOUR CIRCADIAN TYPE

We all have a natural sleep window, or circadian phase, of when our bodies get our best sleep. Learning what sleep window you naturally prefer, based on your circadian type, will be incredibly helpful in understanding your sleep picture and it will help you create realistic goals.

There are three typical circadian types: neutral, morning larks, and night owls. *Neutral* circadian types are the most common. This cycle rises at 6:00 or 7:00 a.m. and rests by 10:00 or 11:00 p.m. While their window may fluctuate a bit, it generally stays in that vicinity.

Morning larks are people who have a natural propensity to go to bed earlier and rise earlier, rising at 2:00 or 3:00 a.m. and sleeping by 6:00 or 7:00 p.m. These types may have some difficulties staying awake at parties but are bright-eyed and bushy-tailed early in the morning when others are still sleeping.

Night owls are those who stay up late and get up late; rising at 9:00 or 10:00 a.m. and sleeping at 1:00 or 2:00 a.m. Many people have probably heard of a "night owl," someone who likes to stay up later, but may not know that it is a naturally occurring phenomenon related to circadian phases. It often carries an underlying assumption that the person has the ability to easily change his or her schedule to a "normal" schedule, but chooses to be lazy. Unfortunately, it can create unrealistic expectations for true night owls who actually have quite a difficult time trying to shift their schedules earlier due to the strength of the natural biological drive to maintain that sleep window.

Night owls often have more difficulties than morning larks in part because their peak energy and focus match up poorly with the structure of the greater social environment. Most night owls work on "normal" 8:00 a.m. to 5:00 p.m. schedules, which can cause some difficulties because a night owl naturally won't get tired until later but will still have to wake up early for work. This often leads to a repeating cycle of several nights of sleep deprivation followed by a night of "catch-up sleep" due to the buildup of sleep appetite before another few nights of sleep loss. There is also research that suggests that having a delayed circadian phase is associated with increased risk for depression, suicidal thoughts, and alcohol and drug use. This is not to say that night owls are doomed to poorer outcomes. Rather, it speaks to the importance of listening to our natural rhythms so we can be more realistic about moving at a realistic pace.

Knowing our baseline sleep window gives us an idea of where our best sleep naturally occurs. This works well if your natural sleep window matches with your desired sleep schedule. However, there is often at least a small mismatch. In these cases, it can be helpful to start with your natural sleep window and gradually shift toward your desired sleep schedule. This process can be done in a sustainable fashion by shifting your schedule by 15 to 30 minutes each week. Any greater or faster does not give all of the bodily clocks enough time to catch up and can cause your sleep to snap back to the undesired schedule.

Identifying your natural sleep window can be a little tricky, but with two weeks of sleep log data, general patterns of when you naturally feel sleepy and naturally wake up should start to appear. If you are not feeling sleepy until midnight or later on a regular basis, you may be a night owl. Conversely, if you just can't seem to stay up until 8:00 p.m., you may be a morning lark. Whatever your propensity, keep it in mind as you start scheduling your sleep.

EXERCISE: MY NATURAL SLEEP WINDOW

Rise Time
If you didn't have any pressures from the outside world, when would you naturally wake up and get out of bed?

____:_____

What time are you currently getting out of bed?

____:_____

Time difference between natural and current time:
_____ hrs

Bed Time
If you didn't have any pressures from the outside world, when would you naturally feel sleepy enough to fall asleep within 30 min?

____:_____

What time are you currently going to bed?

____:_____

Time difference between natural and current time:
_____ hrs

Circadian Type

I naturally identify as: Morning Lark   Neutral   Night Owl

My sleep log shows: Morning Lark   Neutral   Night Owl

My work schedule shows: Morning Lark   Neutral   Night Owl

Sleep Schedule Gap

Taking a look at your bed and wake times above, how closely does your *current* sleep schedule align with your *natural* sleep schedule?

Rise Time:	Within 1 hrs	Within 2 hrs	More than 2 hrs
	Healthy	*Variable*	*Unhealthy*
Bed Time:	Within 1 hr	Within 2 hr	More than 2 hrs
	Healthy	*Variable*	*Unhealthy*

Do I need to shift my schedule?   Yes   No

ESTABLISH A CONSISTENT SLEEP SCHEDULE

Knowing our natural propensity for when we want to sleep is a helpful starting point to inform our sleep schedule. For many of us, there is often a resistance to establishing a time for going to bed and a time for waking up. Perhaps we feel like the rigidity imposes on our sense of freedom. Perhaps it's a residual response from when we had mandated bedtimes as kids. Now that we're adults, can't we can go to bed whenever we want? Well, yes. But consistency serves us all, regardless of age.

Setting and following bed and wake times lies at the heart of a healthy sleep practice. This regularity reconditions our bodies and minds to be alert during the day and relaxed at night. Establishing your sleep framework will allow you to recalibrate, move out of your disrupted sleeping pattern, and increase your performance throughout the day. Let's take a look at how we can figure out what times work best for us.

Set Your Rise Time

We begin with "anchoring" our day with a consistent rise time. As a general rule, it is best to pick one time that works for every day of the week, including weekends. This usually is very unpopular among my clients because it means no more sleeping in on weekends. But while we are resetting our sleep, this is a very important piece to hold firm to because it restores routine and builds our sleep appetite consistently each day. For clarification, our rise time is when we get out of bed; our wake time is when we wake up. Ideally we want them to be the same, but for those who have a tendency to stay in bed after waking up, whether reading the news or lounging, the rise time may be much later.

To identify a time, take a look at your sleep log data from the past one to two weeks. You should be able to quickly spot a range for your bed and wake times. If you don't, there's an exercise at the end of this segment to help you find one.

Set Your Bed Time
Once you land on a wake-up time that feels comfortable for you, you can choose your ideal bedtime. First, take a moment to assess how many hours of sleep per night leave you feeling at your best the next day. Use the data you've collected from your sleep log, sleep story, or circadian type. Many people tend to gravitate toward 8 hours due to the influence of media, or friends and family, but make sure to choose a time that is best for your own particular needs. Remember, the better able you are to tune into your own specific needs, the more likely you will be able to sustain consistent quality of, and satisfaction with, your sleep.

Most people would love to fall asleep immediately upon lying down, but unfortunately we operate more like a dimmer switch than a power button. Subtracting your desired hours of sleep per night from your rise time will almost get you to your desired bedtime but does not account for the time it takes you to fall asleep. To do this, you add an additional 30 minutes to your ideal amount of sleep. For example, if you feel best after seven hours of sleep and identify a 7:00 a.m. rise time, your ideal bedtime would be 11:30 p.m.

Adhere To Your Schedule
Establishing and adhering to a consistent sleep schedule capitalizes on our natural propensity to develop routines.

This includes no sleeping in on weekends, which reduces your sleep appetite for the following night (by waking up later in the day) and exposes your body to jet lag (by delaying your wake and sleep rhythms). Despite how good it feels to sleep in on a Saturday or Sunday, you will be setting yourself up for another sleep-deprived week, starting with an exhausting Monday.

Changing one's sleep schedule sounds easy and looks simple on paper, but it often takes deliberate intention and effort to implement, particularly when social activities, movies, work, and travel beckon you to make exceptions. It is often challenging to break this habit, so rewarding yourself with something small for each week that you maintain your prescribed sleep schedule can also help motivate you. As your sleep regulates again, it will create a stabilizing inertia that will keep your sleep on track in the future even with periodic fluctuations to your bed and rise times (i.e., plus or minus one hour).

What I often find with my clients is that if they've stayed up too many nights, they like to play "catch up." *If losing sleep is so bad for my health, shouldn't I make it up as soon as possible?* Normally, if we lose a few hours of sleep before a presentation and go to bed a bit earlier the following night, our bodies can adjust and restabilize our sleep-wake rhythms. This practice works great for many people throughout their lives. However, making this a habitual pattern can cause your sleep to become unstable and ultimately work against you.

....

EXERCISE: CALCULATING YOUR SLEEP SCHEDULE

....

1. Find your new TIB:

   Your Optimal Amount of Sleep   _____ hrs

                                    +   30 min

   New Time in Bed (TIB)*:   =   _____ hrs

2. Set your new "anchor" time to start your day:

   New Rise Time (RT):   ____:_____

3. Calculate your new bed time:

   Input New Time in Bed (TIB):   –   _____ hrs

   New Bed Time (RT-TIB):   =   ____:_____

*From your sleep log

SET AN INTENTIONAL ROUTINE

The routines we inhabit between our wake time and our bed time significantly influence our progress in following our sleep schedule. Developing a morning, daytime, and bedtime routine that intentionally aligns with our optimal sleep times will be vital.

Morning Routine

Waking up on the first few mornings of your prescribed sleep schedule can be rough. You may feel more sleep inertia than usual so it is important to set up some activities to help energize and activate you as quickly as possible to reduce the duration of the grogginess and reset your body's circadian clock. Choosing activities that are stimulating but not too aversive can take some experimenting. I generally try to get people to think of activities that will engage them in physical, social, and environmental domains.

Physical domains can include exercise, showering, drinking water, and eating food. As you can imagine, these activities can help start your metabolism, raise your heart rate, and raise your body temperature, all of which signal to your body that it is time to be awake. Exercise is a popular choice and can be as simple as a push-up or walking to the front door and back.

After identifying a few physical activities, picking some social activities will help us diversify our choices. In this age of interconnected technology, phoning or texting a friend or family member is quite popular. The purpose of including social activities is to activate more complex neural connections typically used when awake. While sleep itself is a very dynamic period of brain activity, engaging in small talk with your partner, children, or friend upon awakening provides another circadian cue for awakening.

Figuring out some ways to use environmental cues to help us wake up can energize us. You may remember that light is the most powerful alerting cue, which is perfect for your morning routine. Turning on our bedroom lights and opening our blinds immediately, even when it is cloudy outside, will expose our circadian clocks to bright light and help awaken our bodies for the day.

Implementing as many of these morning activities works best when you get out of bed immediately, which means eliminating the beloved snooze button. Using the snooze button in the morning fragments your sleep and can lead to feeling more tired rather than more rested. Getting out of bed quickly will reduce our sleepiness quicker, prepare us for the day, and start building our sleep appetite for the following night.

Daytime Routine

During the day, we naturally oscillate between waves of focus and fatigue. This biological movement is the same ultradian rhythm our sleep moves through, just in reverse. When we sleep, we move from light sleep to deep sleep; when we're awake, we move from high energy to low energy. Working in concert with this natural rhythm allows us to work smarter. That can translate to scheduling project sprints when our energy is cresting and scheduling periodic breaks when our energy is waning.

The timing of these rhythms differs depending upon your natural circadian cycle, but in general, people tend to feel most focused between 9:00 a.m. and noon. This can be a great time for tasks that require clear focus and concentration. After lunch, there is a natural dip in your alerting signal from 1:00 p.m. to 3:00 p.m., which can be an excellent time for a brief nap or exercise (we will explore this more in Chapter 9). Lastly, there is another spike in alertness between 6:00 p.m. and 9:00 p.m., which is followed by a rapid drop in energy. This coincides nicely with bedtime, so using this natural slide can help you fall asleep quickly and stay asleep through the night.

Nap Time

Naps implemented in the correct manner and at the right time of day can actually be helpful. Taking a nap before 2:00 p.m., 10 hours before bedtime, and keeping it under 30 minutes can actually be quite beneficial as a quick cognitive rejuvenation early in the afternoon. However, stay out of your bed the rest of the day; remember that we don't want to associate it with anything except sleep and sex. Other forms of recharging throughout the day can be exercising, socializing, and eating. When we are unable to recharge, we can continue to work productively but often below our best, similar to a car running on fumes. If you're interested in exploring more of the benefits of peak daytime performance, check out the Recommended Resources section.

Bedtime Routine

As our bodies' natural rhythms slow down at dusk, establishing a calming bedtime routine, or bedtime buffer, can help ease our minds and bodies into sleep. This 30- to 90-minute window before our bed times creates a smooth transition between the demands of work or home life and sleep. This buffer zone so often becomes blurred as we tell ourselves that we can answer one more email, watch one more show, or socialize for 10 more minutes. These activities can be innocuous for some, so it's important to be honest with yourself when distinguishing relaxing activities from those that may hook your attention.

Buffer Time

Start with identifying the amount of buffer time you need. I generally recommend at least 60 minutes because it gives us enough time to really separate our active minds and bodies from our resting, sleeping states. An hour can sound like a lot of time at first, but it fills up quickly once you start adding things to it, such as brushing your teeth, washing your face, setting up for the next day, and changing into pajamas. If it sounds too daunting, you can try 30 minutes at first and slowly work your way up to 60 minutes as you feel more comfortable. (If you have trouble falling asleep after bedtime, try getting out of bed for a brief period.) The exercise at the end of this chapter guides you through the approach.

Once you decide which amount sounds most realistic, add it onto your prescribed bedtime. For example, if you plan on going to bed at 11:30 p.m. and want to use a

60-minute bedtime relaxation window, you would plan on finishing activating activities by 10:30 p.m. Many people find it challenging to start their bedtime routine, so setting a nighttime alarm to remind you to start winding down can be quite helpful.

With the remaining time in your bedtime buffer, be intentional about choosing rewarding and relaxing activities to help you wind down. Some people like to chat with their partner, children, or housemates during that time. Others listen to or play relaxing music, enjoy a star-studded sky, or meditate. Choose what works best for you.

Screen Time

One of the most common questions I get is around screen time during our buffer window. Based on what we know about the stimulation by both the light and content of electronic devices, I recommend eliminating screens for this zone. This frequently disappoints many of us, myself included, because this could be the only time we can catch up on movies or shows. Conversely, these activities can serve an important purpose in relaxing us, so be honest with yourself and make your best judgment.

If you use your screens to relax and have no problems drifting off to sleep when you go to bed, there is no need to change it now. If, however, you find it difficult to fall asleep after using your screens, you may want to try an experiment by replacing it with a different activity for a week and see if you notice any differences. If this second scenario happens to you, remember that it is only temporarily more stringent to help anchor a healthy sleep practice. Continuing your good sleep practices after this reset will help you maintain your restful sleep and likely allow you to introduce a little flexibility into your routine without getting pushed too far off course.

....

EXERCISE: BUILDING MY ROUTINE

....

This brief exercise will help you illuminate your current morning, daytime, and bedtime routines. Take a few moments to identify how many strategies you currently use.

New Wake Time   ____:_____

Morning Routine

Bright Light	None	Sometimes	Daily
Physical Movement	None	Sometimes	Daily
Breakfast	None	Sometimes	Daily
Social	None	Sometimes	Daily
_____	None	Sometimes	Daily

What I'm doing well:

_____

_____

What I'd like to do better:

_____

_____

Daytime Routine

Work Sprints	None	Sometimes	Daily
Regular Breaks	None	Sometimes	Daily
Lunch	None	Sometimes	Daily
Nap	None	Sometimes	Daily
Exercise	None	Sometimes	Daily
Dinner	None	Sometimes	Daily
_____	None	Sometimes	Daily

What I'm doing well:

_____

_____

What I'd like to do better:

_____

_____

Bedtime Routine

Nighttime Alarm	None	Sometimes	Daily
Dim Lights	None	Sometimes	Daily
No Screens	None	Sometimes	Daily
Relaxing Activity	None	Sometimes	Daily
Cleansing Rituals	None	Sometimes	Daily
Next Day Prep	None	Sometimes	Daily
_____	None	Sometimes	Daily

What I'm doing well:

_____

_____

What I'd like to do better:

_____

_____

New Bed Time _____:_____

Adding one strategy that you are not currently doing "Daily" during each time of day will help your body more clearly differentiate wake from sleep. Developing these clear distinctions are powerful tools that can benefit anyone, from those with minor sleep disruptions to those who suffer from insomnia.

STRATEGIES FOR INSOMNIA

Insomnia, contrary to popular belief, can affect all of us. It can range from a brief spell like a couple nights of jet lag after an overseas trip, to a chronic problem such as a few years of sleepless nights after a traumatic loss. What makes insomnia so frustrating is that we will have the time to sleep but will have difficulties falling or staying asleep. Learning how to change this problem begins with understanding how it arises.

Arthur Spielman, a pioneering figure in sleep research, defined a seminal model for how insomnia often develops: a stressful event disrupts our sleep and causes us to try to compensate for lost sleep unsuccessfully, leading to worries about getting more sleep, which eventually develops into a self-sustaining difficulty with sleep.

Once it becomes self-sustaining, how do we intervene? There are a few methods for breaking that cycle, but the most commonly used path starts by temporarily adhering to a regular sleep schedule.

For example, one of my clients recalled that his sleep problems began a few years ago when he stayed up to finish a project for work. Exhausted, he went to bed early that night and got more sleep, but then had difficulties falling asleep the following night. Getting less sleep that night caused him to feel more tired the next day and led him to try to go to bed earlier to make up for lost sleep. "It worked before so it should work again," he thought to himself. This time, however, he did not fall asleep right away. Instead, the memory of feeling tired after the previous incident of lost sleep popped into his head as he tried to sleep. Despite feeling exhausted, he ended up lying awake in bed feeling frustrated that he was not falling asleep. Several nights of this unpredictable sleep eventually led to a growing anxiety about getting sleep.

Consolidating Sleep (Sleep Restriction and Sleep Compression)

When we reach the point where it consistently takes us longer than 30 minutes to fall asleep, our bodies and minds are beginning to associate the bed and bedroom with being awake or in a state of "anxious awareness." This negative association with your bed can happen quickly, so replacing that pattern with a more positive experience is crucial.

So how do we unlearn those harmful associations? This happens in a two-fold process. The first step is applying stimulus control, or reducing the number of things associated with the bed (e.g., thinking about to-do lists, watching TV, working on your laptop, answering emails on your phone, etc.). Weakening these associations may take a few weeks, so in the meantime, you will also be strengthening your body's association between sleep and your bed. To do this, you can either do sleep compression or sleep restriction. Both require you to continue to track your sleep and to pay attention to your sleep efficiency (SE). If it is taking you longer than 30 minutes to fall asleep or you find yourself awake at night (WASO) for more than 30 minutes, your SE is probably approaching 80%, which is the threshold for applying either sleep compression or sleep restriction.

Sleep compression requires that you shorten the amount of time you are in bed by 15 to 30 minutes each week by going to bed later by that amount and waking up at the same time each morning. This process gradually reduces your sleep opportunity, or the amount of time you have

available to sleep until you are spending a greater proportion of your time asleep while in bed (i.e., increasing your
SE). As you shorten your sleep window, continue to keep
an eye on your sleep efficiency. As long as your SE is below
80%, you will continue to compress your sleep by another 15
to 30 minutes each week until you are spending at least 80%
of your time asleep while in bed. After your SE reaches 85%,
you can then slowly increase your sleep opportunity by 15
to 30 minutes as long as your SE stays above 85%.

Sleep restriction uses the same principles as sleep compression but on a faster time scale. The difference is in the
reduction of your sleep opportunity. In sleep restriction, you
add 30 minutes to your total sleep time (TST) and use that
as your structure for your sleep schedule. For example, if
you are sleeping only 6 hours per night but are in bed for
8 hours, you would restrict your time in bed to 6.5 hours
per night. As usual, you would use your rise time as your
anchor point and determine your bedtime from there. Using
the above example, if your rise time is 7:00 a.m., you would
wait until 12:30 a.m. to go to bed. This drastic reduction
in the amount of time you can spend in bed works to con-
dense your sleep by causing you some sleep deprivation
in the short-term. The idea is that you will fall asleep more
quickly and stay asleep due to the mild sleep loss, which is
in fact what we see in the research and in clinical practice.
Once your SE is above 85%, you can then increase your
sleep opportunity by 15 to 30 minutes each week, just like in
sleep compression.

If, however, you are sleeping an average of five hours or

less per night, it is not recommended to reduce your sleep opportunity below 5.5 hours. Restricting one's sleep below 5.5 hours per night on a regular basis can be dangerous and more harmful than good. Limiting yourself to only 5.5 hours of time in your bed should quickly amplify your sleep drive and help you consolidate your sleep. You will feel very sleepy and tired, so if you fall into this category, I would definitely recommend consulting with a professional to help support you through this process.

As you can see, this method is more challenging to manage than sleep compression due to the noticeable effects of sleep deprivation initially created by restricting your sleep. It can be more difficult to adhere to this schedule and be dangerous if you need to drive long distances during the day or for the reasons stated above. Thus, it is usually recommended that you work actively with a trained sleep professional knowledgeable in implementing and monitoring sleep restriction safely. Sleep compression may trigger some adverse health conditions and should also be used with caution and ideally in consultation with a trained professional.

Sleep restriction may not be recommended for people who are at risk of falling or those who have a family history of seizure disorders, bipolar disorder, or other sleep disorders (including obstructive sleep apnea). Purposefully restricting one's sleep may trigger these health risks so it is always a good idea to check with a professional before jumping right in. If you have any doubts, please consult with a sleep specialist before implementing sleep restriction.

Insomnia & Napping

Napping for many people can be a very enjoyable endeavor. When work is done, chores are finished, and the sun is filtering down onto the couch, why not soak in the warmth for a snooze? However, for those with insomnia, naps can actually add to their difficulties sleeping. Ideally, consolidating our sleep at night will satiate our need for sleep during the day and prevent the need for a midday nap. Staying active during the day will also help us build the necessary sleep drive so we feel sleepy again at bedtime. If, however, we use some of that sleepiness during the day by taking a nap, our sleep drives may not be strong enough by bedtime to fall asleep.

The end result is that we will fall asleep later when our sleepiness finally achieves threshold levels; our sleep will then be truncated because we have to wake up at the same time in the morning for work, which then creates an even greater desire to take a nap the next day. Seemingly innocuous at first, this can quickly become a vicious cycle and leave one perpetually underslept and chronically tired.

Worry Time

Scheduling "worry time" is not traditionally considered a core aspect of sleep therapy, but since worry and anxiety can occur frequently while trying to shift sleep patterns, I believe it is an important aspect to include. As sleep becomes increasingly more difficult to obtain or seemingly out of our control, it is natural to start feeling somewhat anxious about it.

We often experience anxiety or spend time worrying about things right when we are trying to fall asleep. Some of these thoughts are helpful, such as trying to remember an email you need to send in the morning or groceries you need to pick up on the way home from work. However, these helpful reminders tend to linger despite our best efforts to push them away. So what should you do with these thoughts? A helpful method for hanging onto the useful ones at a more appropriate time requires a piece of paper and scheduling 10–20 minutes earlier in the day (at least 2–3 hours before your bedtime) to think about them.

....

EXERCISE: WORRY TIME
....

Write down your various thoughts and worries in one column. Once you have some of them listed, look at each one and write what, if anything, you can do about it in the adjacent column. If you cannot think of anything, write, "Nothing at the moment, and I'll take a look tomorrow." Then so on. After you write something down for each thought or worry, fold the piece of paper and set it aside. This physical action helps your mind set these thoughts aside so you can stop thinking about them. If one of those thoughts pops into your head at bedtime, reminding yourself that you already took care of it during your worry time will help your mind relax and let it go. Here's an example you can use:

Worries	**Next Step**
What I'm worried about	What I can do about it

This task may sound a bit elementary, but it is actually a very effective exercise. We are complex social beings who understandably have to juggle a lot of responsibilities. Even with the myriad tasks we have to accomplish, our minds are able to focus on work while at work, family while with family, and leisure when having fun. Thoughts from other domains wander in periodically but in general, we train our minds to stay focused during those designated times and they learn to do it beautifully. Thinking about to-do lists or worrying about various problems may seem less controllable when they surface at night, but such thoughts are in actuality just as trainable. Giving yourself permission to acknowledge these thoughts at a regularly scheduled time allows them to exist at a time that works for you and lets you get some sleep.

This strategy worked beautifully for a student I worked with. She came to the college counseling center frustrated that her mind seemed perfectly fine during the day but became very active the moment she tried to fall asleep. *My thoughts rush into my mind the moment I go to bed, and then I can't shut my brain off.* She had tried meditation to "clear her mind" but stated that it did not seem to work for her. As an organized, motivated, and high-achieving person, this was frustrating because she was able to think her way through many of the challenges she was faced with but could not think her way to sleep. She could recognize the thoughts as sleep disruptive in the moment, but trying to stop thinking about them just made the thoughts more persistent. Instead of her trying to stop the thoughts, I suggested that she think about them as much as she wanted but at a specific, structured time during the day by intentionally scheduling worry time. It sounded quite basic to her at first, but she agreed to try it anyway. After the third week of practicing this strategy, she remarked that her thoughts and subsequent irritation at bedtime died down significantly as the thoughts seemed to remain in that daily timeslot. When they did poke out at bedtime, she was able to get them down in her journal and leave them there until the next day.

I include this case example because I think it illustrates some important aspects of this exercise. Many people, like this student, feel skeptical about scheduling worry time at the beginning. It can be difficult to fully believe that it will be helpful before experiencing it. It also requires them to commit to trying it for a period of time. Despite her skepticism, her openness to trying it allowed her to test it long enough to evaluate if it was actually helpful or not. And, similar to her, most people who decide to try this exercise are pleasantly surprised at how quickly their minds learn to keep thoughts and worries to a time they designate. In Chapter 7, we will delve into additional practices that can also help calm your mind and body.

....

EXERCISE: TROUBLE FALLING ASLEEP
....

When we have trouble falling asleep, the age-old saying is to count sheep. A more science-backed approach is actually getting out of bed for a brief period. Here's how to do it:

- Get out of bed if you are not falling asleep within 20 minutes, either at the beginning of the night or if you wake up in the middle of the night.

- Go to another room or area within your bedroom and do a calming or relaxing activity until you feel sleepy enough to try to fall asleep again.

- Return to your bed once you feel sleepy again.

These instructions often give people pause because few people want to get out of bed at night. It requires some trust that the technique will actually work. To help you follow through, it also requires thinking of activities you can do in this situation beforehand. Applying the implementation intention framework to these instructions can be very helpful in successfully adhering to stimulus control. The following exercise will guide you through this process:

Take a moment to write down a few possible activities that you can do that are calming, relaxing, and potentially boring (e.g., reading a nonstimulating book, listening to music or a guided meditation, knitting, folding laundry, washing dishes, coloring, etc.). Be creative and realistic.

- Pick a place in your home where you will do these activities. Ideally, this will be outside of your bedroom, but if not, a place that can feel separate from your bed.

- When you have selected a nice spot, spend a little time making sure to leave the necessary materials there (e.g., the book) and make it comfortable. At the UC Berkeley Sleep Clinic, one of the therapists described this as "creating a nest." I loved this description because it brought a fun and comforting association to this exercise.

- Lastly, take a few moments to imagine yourself going to this designated relaxation spot.

Stimulus control is a powerful tool to help you sleep but can be challenging to implement consistently. Hopefully, combining it with the implementation intention exercise will

support you in strengthening your body's association of
being in bed and sleeping.

PUTTING IT ALL TOGETHER

Here is a list of the sleep strategies covered in this chapter
for quick reference.

- Identify your circadian type: this will be your starting point
  if you want to change your regular sleep cycle.

- Establish a consistent sleep schedule: set a rise time and
  bed time to anchor your sleep and wake cues for
  the day.

- Establish a morning routine: activate your physical, social,
  and environmental cues.

- Establish a daytime routine: take regular short breaks
  every 60–90 minutes.

- Establish a bedtime routine: implement a 30- to
  90-minute bedtime buffer.

- Sleep consolidation: consolidate your sleep through either
  sleep compression or sleep restriction if your are working
  with a behavioral sleep medicine specialist.

- Scheduled worry time: schedule a regular 10–20-minute window at least 2–3 hours before bedtime where you write down your thoughts and what you can do about them.

- Strengthen the bed-sleep bond: get out of bed if awake for longer than 20–30 minutes and stay out of bed when not sleeping.

It can be tempting to try them all at the same time. However, even in the structured environment of sleep therapy, I wouldn't expect someone to start implementing all of these at once in the first week. Implementing the sleep-related strategies covered in this chapter can take time and practice, so please remember to be kind to yourself if you are unable to achieve your goals as quickly as you initially planned. After you become confident consistently applying one or two techniques, add one or two additional strategies each week. In the next section, we will help you build your sleep practices over the course of eight weeks.

"My actions are the ground upon which I stand."
  —Thich Nhat Hanh[5]

PART THREE

SLEEP IN ACTION

The first two sections of this book discuss the myriad ways that sleep affects our lives, provide tools to help us identify our current sleep patterns, and present methods to help us begin improving our sleep. Now that we are equipped with this foundational knowledge, the rest of our journey will be dedicated to integrating this information into our daily rhythms—exercise, nutrition, mindfulness— through incremental behavior changes. Our sleeping lives are inextricably interconnected with our waking lives. The sleeping and wakened states are symbiotic: health and well-being in either state enhances health and well-being in the other. After all, isn't the main point of getting better sleep to feel more vividly alive when we're awake?

Chapter 7

PERFORMANCE: INCREMENTAL IS BEST

Many of the strategies we've discussed for improving sleep performance are based on approaches that deliver effective results within 8 weeks. Two months can feel like a long time in comparison to a more short-term solution like medication, but most people find that if they choose to stick with it, it is a great investment of time and effort. The effects are long-lasting and you will end up with the knowledge and understanding of how to improve your sleep when it becomes misaligned again in the future. Giving yourself eight weeks to establish new routines and stabilize your sleep schedules will typically be enough time to see meaningful, sustainable changes. Even if you see gains within a few weeks, staying with it for the full 8 weeks can only help to solidify your improved sleep and other healthy habits, making them more resilient to change.

Behavior change is challenging; we are physically rewiring the neural pathways of our brains. Not only are we learning a new behavior and forming it into a regular routine, but we are also unlearning an existing habit that we've potentially repeated for years. In this chapter, we will begin to facilitate an intentional and incremental approach, over an 8-week period, that empowers us to successfully implement these sleep strategies through a week-by-week plan.

STARTING WITH WHY

Before we go to what you will do and how you will do it, let's start with why. According to ethnographer Simon Sinek, best known for popularizing the concept of *Why,* "When we communicate our purpose, we communicate in a way that drives decision-making and behavior. It literally taps the part of the brain that inspires behavior."[6]

EXERCISE: WHY I WANT BETTER SLEEP

1. I believe if I can improve my sleep, my life will be:

_____

_____

_____

2. I believe if I can improve my sleep, my physical health will be:

_____

_____

_____

3. I believe if I can improve my sleep, my work will be:

_____

_____

_____

4. I believe if I can improve my sleep, my relationships will be:

_____

_____

_____

SETTING YOUR GOALS

Now that we have a grounding in *why* you want to improve your sleep, the next step is to set specific goals to help you realize them. Seemingly simple steps, such as writing down realistic goals, help us to organize our thoughts toward a focused outcome. Setting goals makes our intentions tangible, helps strengthen our commitment, and gives us a template for successfully achieving these behavioral shifts.

8-Week Challenge Goals

Start with describing the goals you would like to achieve by the end of this 8-week challenge. It can be how much sleep you would like, when you want to sleep by, or how you want to perform. These broad goals set the framework for the next 2 months.

Make Them Measurable

Make sure to frame goals in a way that can be measured. For example, "I want to sleep more" is a little vague, but "I want to sleep for 7–8 hours consistently" can be measured. "I want to feel less exhausted by the end of work" can be modified to "I want to feel refreshed enough to take a walk, 3 times a week, when I get home from work." It is important to identify metrics; they are concrete milestones that make it easy to identify progress and fuel our motivation.

Make Them Achievable

Lastly, reaching goals can sometimes feel daunting at the beginning, especially if you've already accumulated significant amounts of sleep debt. It can be tempting to try jumping from 6 to 9 hours per night on the first day. You're motivated and excited, why not make the change all at once?

The reason is that our brains can only process incremental shifts of 20–30 minutes per week. Trying for anything more is hard to sustain over time and can set you up for failure in the long-term.

A college student I worked with, who typically went to bed around 1:00 a.m., established a challenge goal of going to go to bed at 11:00 p.m. To reach that goal, we set weekly goals: going to bed at 12:30 a.m. the first week, 12:00 a.m. the second week, 11:30 p.m. the third week, and 11:00 p.m. the fourth week. Establishing incremental increases in total sleep over the course of one week established a routine of consistent sleep and built her confidence as she successfully met that goal more often than not.

Conversely, another student tried to jump from a 2:30 a.m. bedtime to a 10:00 p.m. bedtime. He felt like he could make the shift without setting incremental weekly goals. For the first couple of nights, he was able to fall asleep at 10:00 p.m. due to his built-up sleep debt. However, his bedtimes soon began to vacillate between 2:00 a.m. and 11:00 p.m. with seeming irregularity. He grew increasingly frustrated at the process and was ready to give up. After I encouraged him to try shifting in small batches over the course of a few weeks, he began to see more consistent results. Similar to training for a marathon, gradual increases in your sleep schedules will allow your body to adjust instead of shocking your system before it's ready.

To help you get started with crafting your sleep goals, I've provided some common scenarios and goals:

Scenario	Challenge Goal	Weekly Goal
I've got a lot on my plate and just don't have enough time to sleep more; sometimes I'll make it up by sleeping in on the weekends *(insufficient sleep quantity)*	Identify the total amount of sleep per night you want, and set your schedule to allow for that	Increase your sleep amount by 15–30 minutes each week, until you reach your optimal amount
I'm going to bed or waking at different times throughout the week *(inconsistent sleep schedule)*	Based on the amount of hours you want to sleep per night, identify your bed and wake times, and set your schedule accordingly	Increase the number of days you adhere to your consistent sleep schedule by 1–2 days each week
I'm not getting as much done as I used to at work; I feel distracted and unfocused *(suboptimal performance)*	Obtain the optimal amount of hours every day that would allow you to feel rested	Increase the number of days you adhere to your bedtime routine by 1–2 days each week
I'm tired all the time and not able to be fully present with my loved ones *(low-quality connections)*	Obtain the optimal amount of hours every day that would allow you to feel energized	Increase the number of days you adhere to your wake time routine by 1–2 days each week

....

EXERCISE: MY SLEEP GOALS

....

My goals for the next 8 weeks:

1._____

_____

2._____

_____

3._____

_____

My goal for each week:

Week 1: _____

Week 2: _____

Week 3: _____

Week 4: _____

Week 5: _____

Week 6: _____

Week 7: _____

Week 8: _____

PLANNING FOR IMPLEMENTATION

Taking the final step to build out an implementation plan to support each of your weekly goals will help you succeed in reaching them, by retraining your neural pathways. We may have the best of intentions, but we also need to unravel unhealthy habits we've built up.

For example, if your goal in the first week is "I will increase the number of hours I sleep from 7 to 7.5 hours per night," then your implementation plan should outline "when 9:00 p.m. hits, I will start my bedtime routine so I can wake up in time and still get 7.5 hours of sleep." This example identifies a cue (9:00 p.m.) and provides an action you can perform (start bedtime routine) to achieve your goal (7.5 hours of sleep per night) for that week. Though seemingly simple, this kind of implementation plan can make us up to 80% more likely to achieve our desired behavior goals when applied correctly.

Roadblocks

Start by taking your first weekly goal and identify any road-blocks that may prevent you from reaching it. Then plan for how you'll navigate around it. For example, a challenge goal for someone who has trouble falling asleep could be "I want to fall asleep within 30 minutes of going to bed." Then a weekly goal to support that is "I will stay out of bed until bedtime so that my body only associates my bed with sleeping." The *roadblock* is that the bed is a comfortable place to unwind. So the way to navigate around it can be "If I feel tired and want to lie down before bedtime, I will go to the couch instead." This subtle yet deliberate shift will encourage incremental change. Each time you head to the couch instead of your bed, your commitment to this new behavior will strengthen.

A common roadblock to consider is how our new sleep goals make us, or those around us, feel; circadian rhythms and desired bedtimes don't always align with those we are close to. For example, a young professional who is trying to go to bed earlier and feels like he or she is missing out on late night drinks may organize a happy hour instead; an adolescent who discovers that he needs more than 9 hours of sleep per night may have to educate his parents so they can alter homework and dinner schedules; a couple who is trying to stop sleeping in may need to explore morning activities that get them both out of bed. Whether it's our family or friends, discussing and planning for changes at the beginning of the journey are essential. Getting all parties onboard will make the road toward healthy sleep less bumpy and more fun.

Support Team
Finding ways to draw support from those around us is a great way to scaffold our efforts as we advance through this process. First, informing friends and family of our intention to change

our sleep helps garner initial support and build accountability. Second, it opens the space for them to voice their own curiosities and challenges with sleep. Sleep health is a universal topic that is rarely talked about with the same sophistication as exercise or nutrition. Third, sharing our experiences and knowledge of sleep helps us consolidate our understanding of our sleep practice. The old adage that the best way to learn is to teach it to someone else definitely applies here. Lastly, sharing our experiences with others may help encourage them to improve their own sleep health. The essence of establishing a healthy sleep practice is not only how it benefits us, but also how it allows us to be at our best for others.

If you prefer to be more private, then think about sharing your journey with at least one other person. This can be the difference between a short-lived or sustained sleep practice. Familial engagement was a surprisingly powerful motivator for one client I worked with. As part of his morning routine, he called his father who lived across the world as a method for activating his social rhythms. Similar to exercise and nutrition, regular social interaction in the morning hours helps entrain our circadian rhythms. At the end of treatment, he pointed to this activity as one of the most helpful and meaningful because it helped him develop a deeper connection with his father and provided a wonderful reason to continue waking up early each morning.

Reward
We work best when we choose a desired behavior that we want to work toward and reward ourselves incrementally

along the way. If you tell your partner that you will take her phone away unless she stops reading work emails in bed, the likelihood that you will stop that behavior is low. If, however, you say that you will reward your partner with a neck massage if she puts her phone away 60 minutes before bedtime, the chances that she will begin to do that are greatly improved. Both interventions are designed to reduce bright light from entering the eyes late at night and to improve sleep, but the latter creates a positive association with the desired outcome and is more likely to succeed. The more we focus on the positive benefits of sleep, the more we will naturally gravitate toward them.

EXERCISE: MY WEEKLY SLEEP PLAN

Next, set incremental goals for each week. Weekly goals break your challenge goals into manageable, achievable pieces. Be specific on how each week builds on the last. They should be reflective of what you can realistically achieve over the course of a week. When you move into the implementation portion, you may want to revisit and adjust your weekly goals based on your progress.

WEEK ONE   ___ / ___ / ___ to ___ / ___ / ___

My sleep goal for this week is:

_____

_____

My potential roadblocks are:	I'll navigate around it by:
1.	1.
2.	2.
3.	3.

My support for this week is:

_____

My reward for this week is:

_____

WEEK TWO   __ /__ /__ to __ /__ /__

My sleep goal for this week is:

_____

_____

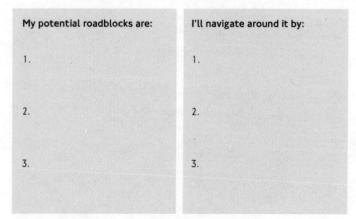

My potential roadblocks are:	I'll navigate around it by:
1.	1.
2.	2.
3.	3.

My support for this week is:

_____

My reward for this week is:

_____

WEEK THREE   ___ /___ /___ to ___ /___ /___

My sleep goal for this week is:

_____

_____

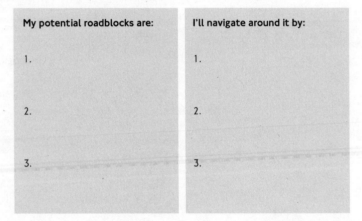

My potential roadblocks are:	I'll navigate around it by:
1.	1.
2.	2.
3.	3.

My support for this week is:

_____

My reward for this week is:

_____

WEEK FOUR   __ / __ / __ to __ / __ / __

My sleep goal for this week is:

_____

_____

My potential roadblocks are:

1.

2.

3.

I'll navigate around it by:

1.

2.

3.

My support for this week is:

_____

My reward for this week is:

_____

WEEK FIVE   ___ / ___ / ___ to ___ / ___ / ___

My sleep goal for this week is:

_____

_____

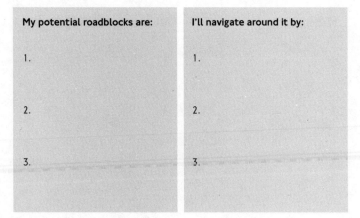

My potential roadblocks are:

1.

2.

3.

I'll navigate around it by:

1.

2.

3.

My support for this week is:

_____

My reward for this week is:

_____

WEEK SIX   ___ / ___ / ___ to ___ / ___ / ___

My sleep goal for this week is:

_____

_____

My potential roadblocks are:	I'll navigate around it by:
1.	1.
2.	2.
3.	3.

My support for this week is:

_____

My reward for this week is:

_____

WEEK SEVEN   ___ /___ /___ to ___ /___ /___

My sleep goal for this week is:

_____

_____

My potential roadblocks are:	I'll navigate around it by:
1.	1.
2.	2.
3.	3.

My support for this week is:

_____

My reward for this week is:

_____

WEEK EIGHT ___/___/___ to ___/___/___

My sleep goal for this week is:

_____

_____

My potential roadblocks are:	I'll navigate around it by:
1.	1.
2.	2.
3.	3.

My support for this week is:

_____

My reward for this week is:

_____

Visualize

After you finish filling out your weekly implementation plan, visualize yourself completing these intentions. It may seem silly, but taking even a few minutes to visualize how you will reach your goal fortifies your commitment to making these changes and can increase your success by up to 80%.

....

EXERCISE: VISUALIZE MY INTENTION
....

- Close your eyes and take a couple of breaths to clear your thoughts.

- Now imagine yourself going through your weekly plan successfully. Try to imagine the details (e.g., the time of day or night, where you are, how you may be feeling, what you may be doing).

- After you complete the sequence in your mind, allow the situation to fade from your mind. Take another breath and slowly open your eyes as you exhale.

PUTTING IT ALL TOGETHER

As we begin to experiment with changing our sleeping pat–terns, the progress we see may not always be linear. In fact, the first week or so of implementing some of the behavioral strategies (e.g., not sleeping in on weekends) can make us a bit sleepier as we regularize our sleep. This is typically short-lived and most people notice the positive benefits even during this period. Even so, this brief increase in sleepiness can deter some people from applying these principles altogether before they have the chance to produce the benefits that they are seeking.

For that reason, it is important to commit to the 8-week challenge. Whether it is learning to play a new instrument, a new language, or programming software, we don't expect to suddenly acquire the skills to play music, speak a foreign language fluently, or write sophisticated lines of code. We intuitively know that we have to set aside an amount of time to learn the new skill. Sleep is the same. Taking one major step each week should be slow enough to allow you to successfully apply new strategies, but fast enough for you to feel like you are making meaningful improvements.

Thich Nhat Hanh once said, "People have a hard time letting go of their suffering. Out of a fear of the unknown, they prefer suffering that is familiar."[7] May these weekly goals give you the space to let go of your old patterns so that you can build new ones that serve a healthier you.

Chapter 8

EXERCISE: LUNGE INTO THE DAY

It is important to note that sleep is just one component of an integrated system of our overall health, not *the* component. Creating a sustainable sleep practice requires a long-term commitment to improving sleep and making healthy choices in several other areas of life. Of the many components of overall health, exercise is one of the most commonly discussed and prescribed behavioral interventions to improve health. Most adults have heard the message "exercise improves your health" at least once in their lives from a doctor, friend, or family member. The truth is that exercise is important to improving our health in innumerable ways: cardiovascular functioning, athletic performance, mood regulation, cholesterol management, and of course, sleep. In this chapter we will cover the relationship between sleep and exercise, as well as practical strategies for building a healthy exercise practice to complement your sleep.

SLEEP IMPROVES OUR PHYSICAL PERFORMANCE

A growing body of research is examining the effects of sleep on physical performance because of the desire to maximize every possible avenue. Research at Stanford provided some of the clearest evidence for the link between sleep and exercise. In the study, collegiate basketball student-athletes were split into two groups. The first half slept their regular 7 to 8 hours per night, while the other half extended their sleep to at least 9 hours per night. Just that extra hour provided amazing performance benefits, including improvements in sprint times, reaction times, and 9% increases in 3-point and free-throw shooting. Studies like this have caught the attention of many athletes in the major sports leagues who now make sleep a priority to help them perform at their elite levels.

The benefits of sleep on exercise definitely extend to the general population as well. Getting enough sleep at night allows our muscles to repair themselves, improves our reaction times, and helps us maintain our muscle tone. Whether it's playing with our children or training for a marathon, having a full tank of sleep will help us increase our stamina for these important activities.

HOW EXERCISE IMPACTS SLEEP

Exercise plays a complementary role in improving sleep. How do we know this? Research with adults has found that regular exercise can help people fall asleep more quickly, decrease nighttime awakenings, sleep for longer periods of time, and even increase their amount of deep sleep. Even into later adulthood, exercise can help consolidate nightly sleep and reduce some of the sleep fragmentation associated with aging.

So, exercise helps us sleep, but how? The obvious inference would be that physical exhaustion somehow adds to our sleepiness and thus allows us to sleep. If this were the case, then all you would need to do is workout until you collapsed midstride on the treadmill, literally running yourself to sleep! Fortunately, the picture is actually more nuanced because who wants to be sweating up a storm at bedtime just to get some sleep?

Part of the relationship between exercise and sleep is related to the circadian clocks located in the muscles. The body's master clock resides behind the eyes in the suprachiasmatic nucleus (SCN) that is most sensitive to light and dark, but there are also peripheral or secondary clocks located in the muscles that are particularly sensitive to exercise. Adding exercise to our regular routines at the beginning of the day activates the peripheral circadian clocks located in our muscles, aligns them with our master body clocks, and helps keep our circadian rhythms in proper alignment. While regularly tuning the clocks in our muscles with exercise is helpful in entraining our sleep, it is not strong enough to regulate our sleep schedules by itself.

Exercise can also impact sleep indirectly by its impact on the circadian rhythms of one's core body temperature. The temperature of our bodies naturally follow a daily cycle, reaching the highest temperature in the early evening and dropping to the lowest trough in the early morning, approximately 2–3 hours before our natural wake times. Doing strenuous exercise can significantly raise our core body temperature and is one way we can accentuate this dip.

When we get vigorous exercise during the daytime, it can influence the body temperature rhythms to help us sleep. Regular exercise has been shown to stretch the body's ability to regulate its temperature as well. If you have a very sedentary life, the contrast between your lowest and highest core body temperatures may be fairly low. If you exercise regularly, you can actually create higher peaks and lower valleys in your core body temperature. For active people, having this greater variability allows for a steeper drop in temperature and facilitates sleepiness during one's normal bedtime. While exercise can be helpful both for sleep and cardiovascular health, overexertion or exercise timed too close to bedtime can actually inhibit one's ability to fall asleep. If you exercise too vigorously too close to bedtime, you run the risk of raising your core body temperature too high or delaying its natural downward progression too long and thus preventing you from falling asleep.

Move Throughout the Week

There is evidence that as little as 5–10 minutes of moderate exercise three or four times a week can improve the time it takes to fall asleep, the average amount of time spent asleep, perceived sleep quality, and mood. Even 30 minutes of walking once a week has been shown to dramatically reduce the likelihood of an early death.

A good minimum benchmark for adults is at least 30 minutes of moderate exercise five days a week (a brisk walk) *plus* muscle-strengthening exercises that target every muscle group at least two days a week (weight-lifting or body resistance exercises such as push-ups). Some people prefer to do their exercise routine more vigorously and quickly, so you can replace the five days of moderate exercise with two to three days of vigorous exercise (jogging, running, swimming) or a combination of both moderate and vigorous exercise.

You can even incorporate the weight resistance training into the moderate or vigorous exercise with circuit training or super sets. The basic idea of this style of workout is to pick a few (3–6) weight resistance exercises that you cycle through in sequence at a pace that maintains an elevated heart rate. For example, if you chose push-ups, sit-ups, and squats as your exercises, you could do four sequences of twenty push-ups, fifteen sit-ups, and twenty-five squats. Another benefit of circuit training is that it builds in the opportunity to work all of your muscle groups in a shorter amount of time.

Those numbers can sound daunting to many people, especially if they have gone several months or years with little regular exercise. However, when you think about the proportion of time you should exercise relative to all activities you will do in a day, it will take up all of 4% of your time.

Lunge into the Day

Knowing that exercise can affect our circadian clocks means that we can leverage the timing of our exercise to improve our sleep. One of the classic methods for using exercise to help our internal clocks differentiate being asleep from being awake and rest from activity is to introduce at least a small amount of exercise in the morning. This could take the form of doing some body resistance exercises (e.g., a couple of push-ups or a few squats), taking the dog for a walk, or even walking to the front door and back. Making this a regular part of your routine will strengthen your wake and sleep systems, especially if you are able to do some of your weekly exercises at this time.

The second way you can use the timing of exercise to help you sleep is to intersperse it in small bites during your day. Based on the basic recommendations for exercise, I tell people that 30 minutes of moderate exercise can be easily broken down into 10 minutes in the morning, 10 minutes at lunch, and 10 minutes after work for five days a week. Taking a short, brisk walk, particularly toward the end of lunchtime, can also be a great way to generate enough energy to counteract the natural middle-of-the-day circadian dip without the need for caffeine or sugar.

Intensify Your Morning Workout

The final component of exercise that can help you sleep relates to intensity. While exercising intensely in the morning appears to consistently have the best benefits for our sleep, it is not always feasible based on our schedules.

Depending on when you are able to exercise, you can adjust the intensity to be most conducive to sleep. Whereas mild exercise regularly dispersed during the day can help with keeping your clocks in tune, moderate exercise in the early evening can have some of the same benefits as vigorous exercise in the morning in terms of helping you fall and stay asleep.

But how is mild, moderate, and vigorous defined? Intensity levels of exercise generally describe how our bodies react to activity in terms of how it affects our heart rate and breathing. Walking a flight of stairs versus running up that same flight will produce different levels of intensity. The same 10-minute jog can be mild, moderate, or vigorous depending on our age, sex, and level of fitness. The following are general guidelines to help give you an idea for how to categorize your exercise:

- Mild exercise is any activity you can do without significantly raising your heart rate or sweating. This includes a slow walk, stretching while sitting at a computer, or playing most instruments.

- Moderate exercise is any activity that raises your heart rate enough for you to begin to sweat. At this level, you can carry on a conversation, but can't sing. This includes a brisk walk, light cycling, or playing doubles tennis.

- Vigorous exercise is any activity that has you breathing hard and fast and has significantly elevated your heart rate above your baseline levels. At this level, you can say a few words at a time, but can no longer carry on a conversation easily. This includes jogging at 6 mph, playing soccer, playing singles tennis, or swimming.

Including these three additional pieces of information—intensity, duration, and time of day—can then help you more precisely determine how these different aspects of your exercise are affecting your sleep. This will then give you greater specificity in adjusting your exercise routines to help you sleep.

ESTABLISHING AN EXERCISE PRACTICE

Establishing an exercise practice to help you sleep will require structuring it in a way that is both realistic and achievable from the beginning. Being specific about the times you will exercise, the types of exercises you will do, and the intensity of the exercise will help you successfully implement your exercise. Setting up the times, exercises, and intensity often takes both creativity and awareness as well. Waking up at 6:00 a.m. to go to the gym may not be realistic if you have been struggling to wake up at 8:00 a.m. However, starting with 3 sets of 10 push-ups when you wake up at 8:00 a.m. could be a more realistic and achievable way to start using exercise to help you anchor your sleep. Likewise, running for three miles three days a week may not be a reasonable starting place if running has not been a consistent part of your physical practice already. Instead, using the elliptical for 10 minutes at a mild to moderate intensity once a week can be a more realistic and achievable place from which you can build.

While there is research stating that vigorous exercise may show the largest benefits for sleep, it's not the place that I begin with my clients nor the place I recommend starting for people looking to use exercise to support their sleep. It has been my experience that starting at an intensity level that feels achievable immediately and achieving it consistently is often a successful method to help anchor your sleep benefit from exercise. As you develop a rhythm, you can then begin to introduce greater intensity into the exercises. We will conclude this chapter with a few brief questions that I like to use to help clients begin to think about how they can start implementing exercise to complement their sleep.

EXERCISE: MY EXERCISE PRACTICE

When using exercise to anchor your sleep, it is often very helpful to do at least a little amount of exercise in the morning shortly after you wake up and during your midafternoon dip to help you get through the day without the need for coffee. As you add exercise to your daily routine, make sure to track the time (date, time of day) and quality (amount, intensity) so you can see the impact it has on your sleep.

After your first week of incorporating exercise into your routine, take a moment to review your progress:

	Type of Exercise (cardio, resistance/ strength)	Amount	Time of Day	Intensity (mild, moderate, vigorous)	No. of Days
Week 1					
Week 2					
Week 3					

Did you notice any differences in how you slept?

_____

_____

_____

Did you notice any differences in your midday energy?

_____

_____

How would you like to adjust the exercise in terms of
amount, timing, or intensity?

_____

_____

Answering these prompts will then help you refine your
exercise practice for the following weeks.

PUTTING IT ALL TOGETHER

Developing a consistent exercise practice is rarely a linear
progression. There are often perfectly reasonable obstacles
that have prevented us from developing a consistent exercise
practice (e.g., increased stress at work, relationships, trying to
change with unrealistic expectations, etc.).

Adding consistent movement to your life is simultaneously often a great practice for self-compassion as it
requires practice, patience, and meeting your body where

it is and not necessarily where you'd like it to be. Acknowledging what you are capable of each week, even if that begins with a 10-minute walk once a week, will set you up for long-term success for your exercise, sleep, and mindfulness practice. This slow and steady approach will get you into a good rhythm as we incorporate an underappreciated domain of sleep health: nutrition.

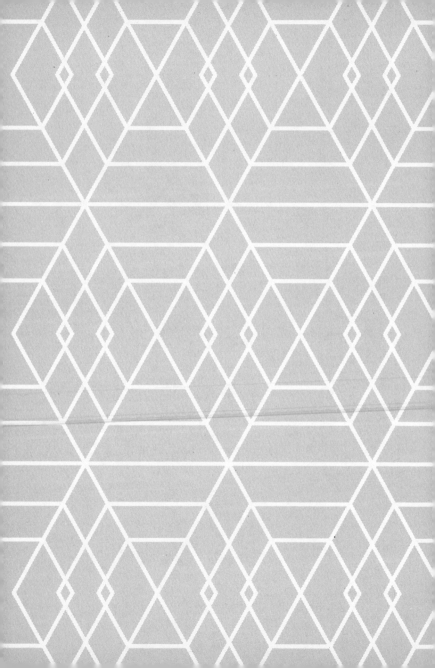

Chapter 9

NUTRITION: BREAK THE FAST

By now we know that our daytime behaviors play a major role in our sleep. What we put into our bodies and when is no different. From the time we eat to the type of foods we eat, these are all factors that affect the efficacy of our organs, the consistency of our sleep-wake schedule, and the quality of our sleep. In this chapter, we will examine how intelligent nutrition choices we make throughout the day can support better sleep at night.

ESTABLISH A REGULAR MEAL SCHEDULE

When we eat serves as a circadian anchor for our sleep. If we eat earlier in the day, our bodies prepare themselves for sleep earlier; if we eat later in the day, our bodies take time to process the food, pushing out our sleep schedules. Each time we eat, we activate several organs that help to process our food. These organs—pancreas, gastrointestinal tract, and kidneys—run on circadian rhythms, meaning they have a time when they function at their best. Our goal is to activate them at their optimal times for eating, which is calorically front-loaded, regularly timed, and not too close to bedtime.

Due to this circadian rhythm and its influence on our sleep, the timing of our meals becomes incredibly important to sleeping well. Regularly timed meals help to maintain adequate energy levels throughout the day and entrain natural circadian rhythms. This consistency keeps our organs' clocks in tune with the body's master clock. It provides another marker for our bodies to differentiate when it's time to eat and be active, or when it's time to fast and rest. Researchers have found this effect to be so powerful that they can change a rat's natural nocturnal lifestyle into diurnal, or daytime, rhythms in just a few days simply by restricting its access to food to the daytime.

This timing translates to eating our largest meal at breakfast, a medium-sized meal at lunch, and our smallest meal at dinner. When we do this, we align our caloric intake with our body's natural metabolic response. When we overeat, it can cause an overactivation of our rest and digest response, or parasympathetic nervous system, and trigger inappropriate sleepiness. This is known as *postprandial somnolence* or, more commonly, a "food coma." Eating regularly timed meals will keep you properly energized and focused during the day so you don't need to take unnecessary naps that can cut into the sleepiness you need to fall asleep at your desired bedtime. Consuming as much as we need at the optimal time keeps us properly energized throughout the day.

ANCHOR WITH BREAKFAST

When we wake up, we will have been without food and water for the longest period of our circadian cycles. By starting our days with a healthy breakfast, we literally *break the fast* by refueling our systems and anchoring our circadian rhythms. Your body is biologically designed to be the most efficient at converting food into energy in the morning. So having your largest meal earlier in the day works in concert with your natural insulin response, which is highest in the morning. Insulin, one of the most important hormones in our bodies, regulates many of our metabolic processes and helps us maintain optimal blood sugar levels.

As the day progresses, our metabolic responses to food switches as our insulin response declines and our glucose response increases. Our metabolic systems are designed to work optimally when we're awake and slow down to conserve energy when we're asleep. The result is that our bodies are less capable of regulating our blood sugar levels the later we eat. Researchers from Harvard found that the timing of a person's largest meal of the day influenced how much weight they lost. Those who ate their largest meals earlier in the day at breakfast lost more weight than those who ate their largest meals at dinner, even when they ate the same amount of total calories. This means that the same donut you had at breakfast would actually be worse for you in the afternoon.

HYDRATE

Water helps us sleep better, as well as feel better throughout the day. It is an essential component of life, and makes up 60% of our bodies, 75% of our muscles, and 85% of our brains. Proper hydration is essential for our brains to function, particularly when they are most active at night. Whether it's consolidating learnings from the day or flushing out toxins, staying hydrated allows our brains to work while we rest.

Without proper hydration, our physical, cognitive, and emotional capacities can break down rather quickly. Chronic dehydration can also cause headaches, dizziness, and muscle weakness. On their own, being sleep deprived or dehydrated are each leading causes of daytime fatigue; together they can make us highly ineffective. The general recommendation to stay hydrated is 8–10 cups or half your weight in ounces of water per day. That doesn't account for other factors, such as high elevation and temperature, where we need more. Also, keep in mind that 20 to 30% of our water intake comes from our food.

EAT COMPLEX CARBS & FIBER

When it comes to what we eat, it appears that it's best to stick with more fiber and more complex carbohydrates, such as legumes, fruits, and vegetables, as well as proteins and healthy fats. These take longer to break down and don't flood the blood stream with glucose, which ultimately yields both short-term and prolonged energy. These won't give you the jolt of simple sugars but will give you the energy to be alert during the day and asleep at night.

The effects of what we put into our bodies on how we feel and function has been a fascinating area of research that has grown rapidly in the past decade. In a recent study at Columbia University, researchers found that the more fiber the participants consumed, the more restorative sleep they got that following night. When participants had higher quantities of processed sugars and simple carbs, such as bread, pasta, and starches, they were more likely to wake up more often than desired and wake up more frequently during the night.

AVOID SWEETS WHEN TIRED

Sleep changes the way that our brains perceive food. If we're sleep deprived, we are more likely to seek out high-calorie foods, such as sugars, simple carbohydrates, and processed foods. That's why the candy jar looks that much more enticing in the afternoon. When we're sleep deprived our body malfunctions across the board: our stomach sends out signals to seek more food than we normally eat; our prefrontal cortex, the part of our brains that regulates our impulse control, is impaired, making it harder to resist that candy; the pleasure centers of our brains become hyperactive, so the candy appears even more enticing than normal; and because our metabolism is slowed, it converts more of those calories into fat. To make matters worse, if we have too little sleep over extended periods of time, we become resistant to the effects of leptin, the satiety hormone. This means that we will start to eat greater quantities of food because it takes more of it to make us feel full. So when you find yourself gravitating toward that pastry, pizza, or donut, it may be that you need to get some rest.

CAFFEINATE EARLY

Sometimes, instead of listening to our bodies and resting when they get tired, we go for the next jolt of caffeine. Coffee, tea, soda, energy drinks, and chocolate are common sources of caffeine that we may consume for pleasure or to gain energy throughout the day. In small quantities it can be fine, even beneficial for some of us, as long as we have it at least 8 hours before going to bed. In larger doses caffeine can cause jitteriness and difficulties with concentration, and it can disrupt our ability to fall or stay asleep. If you regularly consume caffeine, remember to finish your last cup at least 6–8 hours before your bedtime, so that at least half of the caffeine is eliminated from your system.

EAT LESS AT NIGHT

As nighttime approaches, our metabolism slows down in preparation for sleep. When we eat a large or heavy meal close to bedtime, the impact on our bodies is twofold. First, it can misalign our regular sleep-wake rhythms and make it harder to fall asleep and stay asleep. Our digestive system is exerting extra energy to digest at a time when it wants to be resting. Second, consuming more calories than we need will increase the likelihood that we will store those excessive calories as long-term energy stores, or fat.

Conversely, if we eat too little or too far away from bedtime, we still may not be able to fall asleep or sleep through the night. It can be difficult to go to bed hungry, or we may not sleep through the night because we have not gotten enough long-term fuel for our brains to last through the night. This can fragment our sleep when our fuel supplies dwindle and the brain's safety mechanisms alert us to wake up in the middle of the night to refuel.

Finding that ideal window to have our final meal of the day can take a little bit of tinkering. For most of us, it hovers around eating a full meal about three hours before bedtime. Some people may also have a light, healthy snack in between dinner and bedtime, which is a great way to bridge that gap, help quiet our stomach, and allow us to drift off to sleep.

DRINK EARLIER

An alcoholic beverage in the evening can be a nice way for some of us to wind down from the day. These effects can be deceiving. Alcohol, like many sedatives, can allow us to fall asleep quicker and, temporarily, get more deep sleep. We feel like we are sleeping soundly, but as the alcohol metabolizes over the course of the night, our sleep gets lighter and more disturbed. Our REM sleep, the stage that is mentally restorative, becomes significantly reduced. By the time we wake up in the morning, we feel groggy and unrefreshed. So if we drink too much or too close to bedtime, we run the risk of fragmenting our sleep architecture for the rest of the night. The general recommendation for consuming alcohol is to have no more than 2 drinks at least 3–4 hours before bedtime and to have them with dinner.

PUTTING IT ALL TOGETHER

It may sometimes seem like we can't eat anything and everything is bad for us. The main takeaway is simply that we should pay attention to what we put into our bodies. Food and drinks are the fuels that keep our engines and inner ecosystems running, so increasing our intentionality around the types of fuel we provide our bodies will pay dividends on how they function. Additionally, healthy sleep can positively impact how we process the food that we ingest as well as the types of foods that we choose to eat. When we are sleeping well, the timing of our food intake will be optimized to match our bodies' ability to properly use the food that we consume.

There was a lot of information in this chapter. See if you can incorporate any one of these strategies into your weekly goals, and experiment with how it affects your sleep and overall health. Here are some general recommendations for easy reference:

- Consistent meal timing will help entrain your body clocks for sleeping and waking.

- Largest meal at breakfast, moderate meal at lunch, smallest meal at dinner.

- You need at least half your weight in ounces of water per day.

- More fiber plus fewer saturated fats in your diet may increase deep sleep.

- Getting too little sleep will make you feel hungrier and impair your ability to resist junk food.

- Last caffeine at least 6–8 hours before bedtime.

- Last alcohol 3–4 hours before bedtime.

As always, make sure to listen to what your body is telling you about what your need versus what you want.

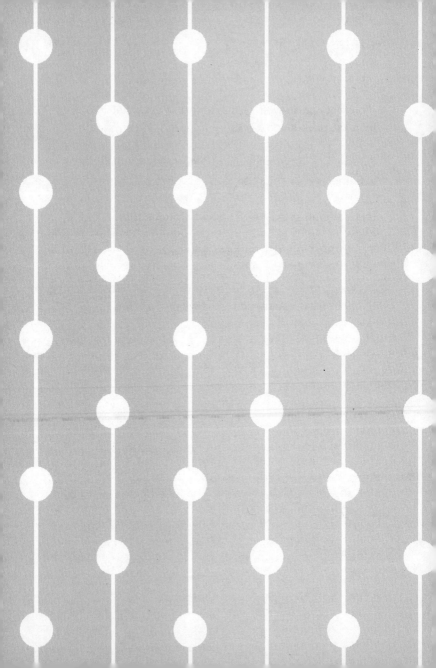

Chapter 10

MINDFULNESS: STRESS LESS

From the science of sleep, we learned how getting healthy sleep helps us manage our stress levels by regulating the sympathetic nervous system. In this chapter, we will examine the symbiotic nature of this relationship in the other direction: how stress affects our sleep. Most of us know from our own experience that stress negatively impacts our sleep, but understanding the physiological and psychological processes involved in stress-related sleep disruption is crucial. Only then can we begin to ask the question, what are the main strategies for managing stress to enhance our sleep?

HOW STRESS IMPACTS SLEEP

We have all experienced times when stressful events disrupted our sleep. The excitement of planning a vacation, anxiety over a deadline for work, or the pain of losing a loved one are powerfully stressful events that can negatively impact sleep by changing both our physiologies and attitudes towards sleep. Training ourselves to notice how our minds and bodies respond to stress tunes our awareness to recognize the signals of stress as they're happening and also informs us how to skillfully address the stress response.

Too Stressed to Rest

Stress is such a visceral experience that it is reflected in some of the most common expressions we have: "my blood is beginning to boil" or "things are getting heated." They all touch upon clear signs of stress: increasing heart rate, feeling flushed or warm, rapid and shallow breathing, and tensing muscles; all signals that the body's initial stress response, or the sympathetic nervous system, has been activated. If the stressor continues, the second component of the stress response, the hypothalamic-pituitary-adrenal axis (HPA), will trigger the release of cortisol to help maintain our physiologic vigilance. Normally, any type of stress we experience will activate the HPA axis to jump-start alertness and prime us to spring into action. In brief instances, this can temporarily push us into insomnia until our stress response recovers. However, when the stressor becomes chronic or if we experience multiple stressors at the same time, our bodies leave the stress response switched on, which does not give us a chance to recuperate. The longer our stress response system remains active, the longer our cortisol levels remain higher than normal, and the more our body temperatures and heart rates are elevated. As we can easily surmise, this creates the perfect recipe for difficulties falling or staying asleep.

My Mind Is Racing

As we learned in the science of sleep, getting healthy sleep is important in regulating our emotions. Without enough sleep, the emotional center of our brains can begin to override the logical center of our brains, leading to greater feelings of anxiety. This anxiety often gets directed toward our sleep or lack thereof. However, worrying about poor sleep the night before often escalates into deep anxiety about tonight's sleep, and even tomorrow night's sleep. Before long, we can find ourselves consumed by recurring bouts of sleep anxiety that increase our sympathetic arousal and decrease the likelihood that we will fall asleep at our desired bedtimes. This progressive anxiety about getting sleep can be quite consuming for many of us. Using relaxation exercises or establishing a regular mindfulness practice is key to rewriting these anxious stories.

ESTABLISHING A MINDFULNESS PRACTICE

It's no secret that relaxation exercises are highly beneficial in rebalancing stress in our lives. They can range widely from simple stress-distraction activities like watching TV to more self-directed mindfulness practices such as meditating. The American Academy of Sleep Medicine includes relaxation exercises and meditation as optional interventions in their guidelines to sleep therapy because they are powerful supplemental techniques even though they have not been shown to significantly improve sleep by themselves. While they all have their usefulness, research shows that a regular mindfulness practice is more effective for sleep than simple relaxation exercises. Whereas relaxation exercises temporarily distract the mind away from sleep-related anxiety, mindfulness practices give us the power to modulate our response to stress.

What Is a Mindfulness Practice?

A mindfulness practice refers to a collection of strategies that help us notice our thoughts, emotions, and behaviors as they are unfolding. As we explored in Chapter 6, increasing our awareness of these elements of our experience is crucial to understanding how they impact the stories we have about our sleep. Each time we are intentionally tuning our attention to our moment-to-moment experiences, we can relax our minds by letting go of stressful thoughts and concerns that we cannot control.

At its core, mindfulness practice allows us to strip away extraneous details and focus on what we are currently experiencing in the moment, without being distracted by thoughts of the future or the past. Mindfulness practice can be done while we are fully engaged in any activity, such as breathing, reading, walking, or soaking in a beautiful sunset. We simply immerse ourselves deeply in the activity, even for a minute or a few seconds, which allows a vast space for calm and clarity to arise. Each of us has experienced these moments of calm and clarity and recalling them gives us motivation to pursue a mindfulness practice. (What's your moment? What does it conjure up?)

Immersive singular focus is in and of itself calming because our brains are not switching to temporally unrelated thoughts. Our brain does not actually multitask (i.e., process multiple competing stimuli simultaneously) even if we perceive or demand that it does. In reality, it switches quickly between tasks, providing the illusion that we are processing them at the same time. While this process can help us juggle different activities, it causes us to miss details, perform the tasks at suboptimal levels, and wear down more quickly. Allowing our brains periodic respites for singular focus reduces excessive strain, generates a sense of calm, and allows our minds to be more at ease as we slip into slumber.

A regular mindfulness practice that brings our attention to the present moment is also particularly useful in alleviating sleep-related anxiety, which is powered by our thoughts of previous poor nights of sleep and projections of future difficulties with sleep. Bringing our senses back to the present moment repeatedly through a mindfulness practice can reduce the cycle of obsessive thinking about past and possible future sleep issues, thereby diminishing sleep-related anxiety.

Mindfulness Practice Facilitates Sleep

Quieting the physiological arousal system can be a significant part of your sleep puzzle. Regular mindfulness practices have been shown to be effective in lowering baseline arousal (process W) during both the day and night. However, the goal of many mindfulness practices is not to make one calm. Rather, the increased feelings of peacefulness are a byproduct of being in the moment and completely present to our experience through letting go of extraneous stimuli and details.

A common example of being ensnared by extraneous stimuli is thinking about work while on vacation. Rather than enjoying our time on vacation, we often think about work we "should be doing" or tasks we may have in front of us when we get back to work. The thinking easily turns into worry, which then manifests as checking emails while lying on a beach, and perhaps being dragged completely back to the work mode from which we had been seeking respite. How maddening that our inability to be in the moment causes us to turn our backs on the recuperative experience we had been seeking and looking forward to: lying on a beach and not worrying about work!

Numerous studies have looked at the positive effects of a regular mindfulness practice. In most of these studies, "regular" mindfulness practice is defined as a daily practice of 20–45 minutes for 8 weeks. Establishing a daily practice of mindfulness has shown to address a wide array of issues from stress, chronic pain, anxiety, depression, and, of course, problems with sleep. The positive effects of a regular practice on our health extend beyond simply improving problems. Research has shown that cultivating a mindfulness practice can also improve happiness, connectedness, optimism, and satisfaction in the workplace.

As powerful results continue to be published showing the effectiveness of regular mindfulness practice in treatment on a macro level, there is also research on how it affects our physiology on a micro level. There is some evidence that having a regular mindfulness practice has a positive impact on both our stress and relaxation responses. Researchers in Thailand found that teaching medical students to employ a mindfulness practice for just four days was correlated to significant decreases in their cortisol levels, the stress hormone. Having a regular mindfulness practice has also been shown to stimulate the vagus nerve, which is part of the relaxation response. The combination of reducing the stress response while increasing the relaxation response is thought to be one of the greatest benefits to good sleep that a mindfulness practice provides. Not only does this help decrease the risk for cardiovascular disease, it will also help us sleep by lowering our stress levels and arousal systems.

A mindfulness practice on a broader level is also a method for heightening the awareness of our senses, thoughts, emotions, and behaviors. Continually bringing our attention to the present moment strengthens our ability to actually recognize when we are engaged in a behavior, thought, or emotion that is nurturing or hindering our sleep. Research shows that we are more perceptive of our thoughts, emotions, behaviors, and environment when we regularly engage in a mindfulness practice. At first, we may only be able to notice it a few times and feel like we are unable to change it at the time. This is normal and perfectly okay. As this skill continues to improve with practice, we will begin to notice more and more of these moments as they are happening. Eventually we will be able to choose to continue to follow the thought, behavior, or emotion down the old familiar paths or pick a novel, more helpful route.

Your Mindfulness Practice

Beginning a mindfulness practice to help us sleep is a fantastic place to start. It is equally wonderful if we only use it while our sleep is offline or if we continue it beyond our sleepless nights. In either case, starting slowly with a small practice will help build it to a level that will serve us in whatever capacity we choose. "Small" can be as little as 1–5 minutes, 1–3 times a week. Many of us can get a bit too enthusiastic when we embark on self-improvement plans and try to jump straight to 30 minutes a day. This is like trying to work out every day after a lifetime of never intentionally getting any exercise. It may feel good the first day or so, but most likely we will quickly burn out. Easing into it with reasonable expectations will engender confidence and self-empowerment each time we are able to successfully practice and establish a sturdy base of consistency that will sustain our practice. For your reference, there are several mindfulness practices in the Resources section that you can choose from. I encourage you to experiment with ones that connect with you.

Once we establish an initial goal, applying the principles of implementation intention will significantly improve the probability that we will meet it: What time of day? Where? How long? What modality? Many people begin by trying their mindfulness practices at night, either during their pre-bedtime buffer zone or as they lie down to sleep. A mindfulness practice at night can definitely help calm the mind and body before bed, which is exactly what we want. Additionally, a mindfulness practice during the day can also help by keeping those baseline arousal systems low, making it easier to be relaxed at bedtime and throughout the night. The following exercise will help guide you in establishing a successful mindfulness practice to help you sleep.

....

EXERCISE: MY MINDFULNESS PRACTICE

....

The one mindfulness practice I want to start is:

_____

Time of day I will practice:

_____

Duration of my practice:

_____

Location where I will practice:

_____

Number of days I will practice each week:

_____

PUTTING IT ALL TOGETHER

The first half of this book addressed methods to directly help
our sleep; while this chapter covered methods that indirectly
help sleep by lowering our arousal systems. The aim was to
explore how some of the basic components of mindfulness
can help us feel calmer and facilitate sleep. Hopefully, a deeper
message was conveyed that cultivating present-moment
awareness is beneficial not only for sleep but for waking life as
well. As we develop a regular mindfulness practice to complement our sleep, the final chapter will reflect on our 8-week
journeys and the resilience it has given us for the future.

Chapter 11

REFLECTION: PRACTICE WISELY

Now that we have spent these past 8 weeks putting these strategies into practice, the last step is to reflect upon the journey we've taken. We often get so caught up in the achievement that we forget to document what we did that was helpful along the way. When we take the time to review how it went, it allows us to appreciate and glean the wisdom from the entire journey: what was most challenging, what was most helpful, and how will we apply these lessons when our sleep gets knocked offline. Research has shown that when facing a health challenge, even if we are able to reduce our symptoms—in this case difficulties falling or staying asleep—our risk of regressing is higher if we fail to take the time to reflect upon how our beliefs have changed from when we first started making the changes.

REFLECTING ON THE STORY

Regular reflection is an integral aspect of both cognitive behavioral therapy and living mindfully. It allows us to fully understand our experiences both in the past and in the present as we are currently experiencing them moment-by-moment. For some, the changes in how they slept before and after applying the steps in this book can be quite notice-able. Their sleep schedules went from erratic to consistent, or their sleep quality went from feeling fatigued to restful. For others, the changes can be slower or erratic depending upon circumstantial stressors or unknown reasons. Either way, it can be useful to look back at your baseline sleep diaries and compare them to your current sleep.

One of the great benefits of maintaining the sleep dia-ries is that it gives you this great data that shows you how far you've come. Even if your sleep does not look the way that you had hoped, most of us who follow the sleep strate-gies can still pick out some positive trends. If you don't see much positive progress, you may still want to look at how your relationship with sleep, or your sleep story, may have changed. And even if the amount of total sleep is roughly the same, the feeling of having more control over one's sleep can be beneficial.

Making these reflections unique and personal will only help us more deeply encode what we've learned about our sleep into memory. At the UC Berkeley Sleep Clinic, we ask our participants to come up with their top five most helpful aspects of sleep therapy before the final session. Instead of having them simply regurgitate the information, we have them pretend that they are either being interviewed for a video endorsement for why sleep therapy can be helpful or teaching what they have learned to a good friend or family member. It creates a fun atmosphere in which they can reflect upon the gains that they have made and provides a positive final association with their sleep education. Whatever mode of expression you choose, sharing it with someone else can deepen that learning for you as well as broaden the impact of what you've found valuable along the way.

....

EXERCISE: MY SLEEP STORY 2.0
....

1. What is my new relationship with sleep? Draw the image that comes to mind.

2. How has my sleep story changed? What am I
   doing differently?

_____

_____

3. What were the top three strategies that helped me?

_____

_____

_____

4. What will I do in the future when my sleep gets
   knocked offline?

_____

_____

BUILDING RESILIENCE

Our sleep, much like our lives, will inevitably run into a
pothole or two—traveling across different time zones, experiencing a life changing event, or even socializing with friends
late at night. Even when we are able to sustain regular

meditative, exercise, and nutritional practices, sleep will most likely fall out of alignment at some point. Planning ahead will help us right the ship quickly when these situations occur.

Maintain Healthy Practices

Maintaining practices of healthy living when we're not in crisis is one great method for keeping sleep anchored when stress arises. It is far easier to establish consistent sleep, daily exercise, healthy nutrition, and a regular mindfulness practice when we are already relaxed versus trying to entrain these rhythms after a stressor enters the picture. Operating within our healthy range for longer periods of time creates the gravity we will need to pull our sleep back into alignment if it gets knocked a bit out of orbit. This can be particularly helpful when unpredictable life stressors occur such as the loss of a loved one or unexpected changes in job status. Depending upon how jarring the stressful event is, some or all of our healthy habits may get temporarily dislodged until the stressor resolves. When this is unavoidable, sometimes the best thing to do is to simply have realistic expectations. For example, just allow for sleep disruption to happen and accept that it may continue for a few weeks or months until the stressor subsides. Instead of worrying about sleep and adding to our frustration, try doing the best that we can with how much sleep we are getting and shift when we are able to get back on our routines.

Anticipate Stressors

Anticipating upcoming stressors can also help us adjust our sleep and wake routines accordingly. As we approach an anticipated stressor, being more intentional about our health practices can help mitigate some of the highs and lows that accompany these large shifts. Being thoughtful about the foods that we eat or drinking another glass of water while traveling for work can help us sleep more soundly and stay energized during the day. If we are traveling, starting to adjust our sleep schedules ahead of time to match the time zone of our destination can be another way to help adjust quickly.

Other stressors, like the welcoming of a new child, can cause sustained declines in healthy sleep that are unavoidable. No matter how much planning you do, sleep deprivation often accompanies such a life transition. A reasonable strategy to manage a situation like this is to try and let go of one's former sleep patterns until the adjustment to the new addition has settled into a new rhythm. In this case, trying to fight something that you may not have power to control will leave you feeling more drained and frustrated and cause the sleeplessness to persist longer than if you adopted a more accepting attitude. Instead, it's helpful to set reasonable expectations that you will probably feel sleepier in the short-term, but know that the sleep loss will only be temporary.

Even when our lives continue along with minor blips in stress, our healthy habits can still start to crumble. This can easily happen to us all. As our practices fluctuate, continuing to attune our awareness to how we feel, behave, think, or perform will remind us of what helps or hinders us. It is easiest to maintain the practices when they are going well, but expecting to keep them there forever is often unrealistic. It is really up to each one of us to determine how much we can tolerate before we truly take notice and decide that we need to take more intentional action again.

Identify Your Warning Signs

Many of the people I work with wait to make adjustments again until they receive hard news from their health care providers that their health has already been significantly harmed. Others may decide to make changes after their relationships have begun to suffer. We all have particular pressure points that will be more sensitive to change. It can be our family, friends, work, diet, exercise, meditation, sleep, mood, performance, concentration, or something else. And often these triggers will move us into action when our health falls out of balance.

Identifying what those are for you early on can be a great barometer to gauge your overall health and give you a starting place to make adjustments. Additionally, other people in our lives can often see when our health begins to slide more quickly than we can. Giving them permission beforehand to give us this feedback is helpful. Let's take a few moments to write down your reference points so that when future stressors arise you can recover from them more quickly.

EXERCISE: MY RECOVERY PLAN

1. What are my warning signs that my sleep is straying off course?

_____

_____

2. When I identify one or more signs, how much leeway
   will I give myself before I intervene?

_____

_____

3. Whom will I accept feedback from?

_____

_____

The great thing about life, and our sleep, is that it will continue to ebb and flow. No matter how hard we try to maintain healthy sleep practices every night, our sleep will eventually fluctuate. Sleep is a lifelong practice. Taking an attitude of acceptance, both when it is steady and when it is disrupted, will allow you to acknowledge these differences as they arise and help you recover quicker.

IN GRATITUDE

His Holiness the Dalai Lama once said, "Sleep is the best meditation."[8] When I think about why I am drawn to sleep medicine, that saying rings true for me. Sleep has been my conduit toward truly awakening and living more fully. Before treating my sleep apnea, my world appeared like the horizon boundary between the Pacific Ocean and the sky as seen from San Francisco on a typical day: you know it's there, but it looks a bit fuzzy through the fog. Occasionally, the horizon line would be crisp, but the next day the mist would roll back in. After treatment, it felt as if the fog had lifted and the days became clearer. I now experience my life fully awake instead of through the cloudy lenses of my fatigued, former self.

My hope is that, with healthier sleep, you are beginning to experience clearer days as well. No matter how big or small your improvements, you have made an immense effort to understand, appreciate, and augment your sleep. This is the ultimate act of self-compassion. Even if you did not achieve the sleep of your dreams, this continual exploration of the factors that contribute to your sleep will serve you long after you've put this book down. I am truly appreciative of our time together and wish you loving kindness on your path. May you know peace; may you be happy; may you be loved; may you be free from suffering; and, most important, may you sleep wisely.

APPENDIX

RELAXATION
EXERCISES

1. BREATHING

This exercise takes just a few minutes and is typically done while seated in a comfortable position or lying down. For those who are new to this practice, it can be helpful to find a quiet place to sit or lie down somewhere other than your bed or bedroom. Even for relaxation exercises, it is best to practice these first outside of your bed so your body associates bed with sleep, not bed with trying to relax. Ideally, this is somewhere you feel comfortable and safe enough to close your eyes without being disturbed or self-conscious of what others may think if they were to walk past you. It is also helpful to commit to a short amount of time (one to five minutes) to try this exercise. There are several free meditation apps that have timers that provide a gentle ring to signal the end of your meditation. Using one of these can help alleviate any curiosity or anxiety about how much you have been meditating and allow you to simply attend to your breath.

When you find a place and time to try it out, reading through the following script will give you an idea of how to approach the exercise:

- As you allow your body to settle into a comfortable position, gently close your eyes and take three deep cleansing breaths.

- Breathe in through your nose and out through your nose. (I suggest breathing in and out of your nose because it slows the breath and allows the lungs to extract more oxygen from each breath. But if you find it difficult to breathe through your nose, feel free to breathe through your mouth.)

- As you breathe in, notice the cool air rushing up through your nose.

- As you breathe out, feel the warm air rush back out.

- Breathe in again, drawing the cool air up through your nose and down the back of your throat.

- As you breathe out, feel the warmth and tension rush back out.

- Breathing in again, feel the cool air rush up through your nose, down the back of your throat, and into the bottom of your lungs.

- As you breathe out, feel the warmth and tension rush back out.

- After taking these three slow, deep breaths allow your breath to return to its normal pace and rhythm. Start to notice the quality of it.

- Is the exhalation longer than the inhalation?

- Is there a brief pause at the top and the bottom?

- Does it feel effortful or effortless?

- At this point there is no need to change it. Simply notice the slow and steady inhale with an easy and relaxed exhale.

- Take two more breaths and as you exhale the second time, slowly
  open your eyes and bring your awareness back to the room.

As your awareness of your breath expands, you will also be able to
change your current physiological experience to a more desirable
state. When we take an in-breath, our heart rate slightly quickens, and
it slows when we breathe out again. You can use a rhythmic increase
and decrease to increase or decrease energy by changing the ratio of
in-breath to out-breath. To increase your energy, take a long inhale followed by a quick exhale. Try breathing in so your lungs are completely
filled with air to a count of eight and breathing out so your lungs are
completely empty to a count of four. Athletes are often seen doing
this if they want to amp themselves up before entering a competition.
Alternatively, keeping a longer out-breath compared to your in-breath
will have the opposite effect and activate your parasympathetic
response. An inhalation followed by a slow and longer exhalation will
slow your heart rate and calm your body and mind. This is a simple yet
effective way to quickly reset and gather oneself.

2. NOTICING YOUR THOUGHTS

This meditation can be done either lying down or seated in a
comfortable position.

- As you settle in, allow your eyes to gently close and turn your attention to your breath. Notice the quality of it: the pace, the depth, and
  the ease of the air coming in and flowing out.

- When you're ready, allow your thoughts to come to the forefront of
  your awareness, inviting all facets of your thinking mind to flow in
  and around you.

- You may notice them trickling slowly by or cascading through your mind—thoughts of the past, plans for the future, or even judgments or critiques of yourself.

- As these thoughts arise, see if you can observe them as they rise and fall without following them.

- If you find yourself following one of these thoughts, you can unhook yourself by simply acknowledging the thought whenever you become aware of it, allow it to gently float away, and return your awareness back to your breath and to the natural ebb and flow of your thinking mind.

- Every time a new or repeated thought captures your attention, repeat this step of acknowledging it, releasing it, and gently return your attention to your breath.

- Take one last breath and as you exhale, slowly open your eyes and bring your attention back to the room.

When you first start this practice, thoughts will continue to probably catch and hold your attention. This is perfectly normal. Once you realize that you have been following a thought, the practice is to just notice it and unhook yourself from the current thought. The main purpose of being mindful is to notice when you are having a thought and return your focus to your breath. If your mind wanders away again, that is okay. Simply notice the thought wherever you happen to catch it, release it, allow it to fade away, and gently return your attention to your breath: the steady and slow inhale, followed by the smooth and easy exhale.

3. MEDITATION OF THE SENSES

This meditation can be done lying down, but I suggest doing it in a seated position to allow sensations to come from all directions without being impeded by the floor. Spend at least 60 seconds with each sense individually while taking one full inhalation and exhalation before switching to another sense.

- When you find a comfortable position, take a couple of deep breaths, gently close your eyes, and allow yourself to settle.

- After the second exhalation, turn your attention to the sounds around you.

- Allow the sounds to ripple over you without reaching out for them and begin to notice the quality of sensations. Some sounds may be sharp or crisp while others may be muted.

- If thoughts begin to attach themselves to these sounds, acknowledge them, allow them to pass, and then gently return your attention to the waves of sounds around you.

- When you're ready, allow sounds to fade as you take one intentional breath. As you exhale, allow physical sensations to come to the forefront of your awareness.

- Notice the different points of contact: your feet with the floor, the softness of the cushion or chair beneath you, the gentle weight of your clothes on your body, the temperature of the air on your arms, or perhaps a gentle breeze across your face coming from an open window.

- You may feel areas of tension or softness or no feeling at all in different parts of your body. Whatever you feel, allow it to be just as it is.

It may be tempting to shift in your seat or scratch an itch, but if you can, simply notice the sensation and impulse and let it gently pass.

- When you're ready, allow the physical sensations to fade as you take one intentional breath. As you exhale, allow your sense of smell to come to the forefront of your awareness.

- As you slowly draw the air in through your nose, notice the quality of the air as it passes up through your nostrils, down the back of your throat, and into your lungs.

- Is the air warm or cool? Heavy or light? Notice as scents of your clothes, food, environment, even your own breath reveal themselves without actively trying to identify or categorize them.

- When you're ready, allow smells to fade as you take one intentional breath. As you exhale, slowly open your eyes and allow visual sensations to come to the forefront of your awareness.

- Try to maintain a steady, easy gaze and refrain from blinking as much as possible.

- Allow shapes, colors, shadows, patterns, textures, light, and reflections to appear.

- If thoughts begin to form and attach themselves to the objects, colors, or shapes in your visual field, acknowledge them, let them drift away, and gently return your attention to what you are actually seeing and not thoughts of what they are.

- When you're ready, allow your visual field to slowly fade as you gently close your eyes and return your attention to your breath. Take two complete cycles of breath, slowly open your eyes as you exhale, and come back to the room.

You may have noticed that some of the guidance within this exercise is similar to that of the breathing and body scan exercises we have already followed. Repeatedly tuning into your senses in familiar ways will help you strengthen these neuropathways and deepen your awareness of your senses and experiences.

4. BODY SCAN

This type of meditation is often recommended to do lying down, ideally outside of bed so you are not falling asleep during it. While that might sound like a great idea, especially in a book helping you with your sleep, I still recommend practicing it on a couch or mat on the floor because the benefits of this meditation go beyond just relaxing enough to fall asleep. Research has shown that the body scan exercise in particular helps you attune to your body—where you are feeling relaxed or tense—both while you are practicing it and during the rest of your day. The awareness you build during the exercise can permeate your whole day.

There are many ways to practice a body scan meditation. Many people find it helpful to have someone guide them through the exercise. This is one of the first meditations in Jon Kabat-Zinn's MBSR or Mindfulness-Based Stress Reduction course, which has helped people suffering from a wide range of ailments from chronic pain to anxiety and sleep disorders. That version is 45 minutes long, but if that sounds a bit daunting, you can always start by trying one that's 5–10 minutes in length as in the suggested exercise below.

- Start by lying down in a comfortable position with your legs straight and arms at your sides and take a few breaths to settle into the rhythm of your breathing.

- After checking in with your breath, begin by bringing your awareness into different parts of your body, starting with the toes of your right foot, moving into the entirety of the right foot, the ankle, the calf, the knee, the upper leg, and finally the entire right leg. Move to the toes of your left foot, and gradually bring your awareness part by part to your entire body.

- When placing your awareness into these areas, try not to move those parts of the body. Instead, simply see if you can notice any sensations of tension or relaxation in the muscles, bones, and tendons.

- Notice the rhythmic pulse of blood pumping through, or the temperature of the air or pressure of your clothes on the skin that wraps around that body part. You may also not have any sensations coming from that area, which is perfectly fine.

- As you send your attention to each area of your body, remember to try to approach it nonjudgmentally. Pain may elicit feelings of irritation, anger, or resentment, which can then intensify or prolong the duration of the pain. If other thoughts or feelings do arise as you notice an area of your body, see if you can acknowledge and release them and gently return your attention to the actual sensations as they are happening from moment to moment.

- Whether you experience sensations or not, just keep sending your attention to that area for a few moments before letting your awareness of that body part fade away and letting the next area come into focus.

- After you have sent your awareness to each part of your body, see if you can bring the entirety of your body into your awareness. Rest in your awareness of all of the sensations in your body (or lack thereof) for a few full cycles of breath.

- When you're ready, take one deep inhalation, and as you exhale, allow your awareness of your body to slowly fade, returning your attention to your breath again.

- Take another deep breath and slowly open your eyes as you exhale.

Though simple, this can be a challenging meditation at the beginning. We spend so much time in our intellectual and thinking minds, it is common for our attention to wander when trying to tune into our bodies nonjudgmentally. This is also precisely why it is important to continue to practice tuning into your body. Whether through this exercise or the exercise in the next section, enhancing your awareness of how your body is actually feeling in the moment allows you to evaluate if it is getting enough sleep, exercise, nutrition, or rest.

5. WALKING MEDITATION

To begin, find an area where you can walk unimpeded for at least 5–10 paces. Whether in a hallway or in a park, I usually recommend that people pick a time and place where they will not feel self-conscious while they slowly walk back and forth. After you have a place picked out, set aside 5–10 minutes.

- Begin by centering yourself with your breath in a standing position. Place your feet about shoulder width apart and stand in a comfortable posture with your weight equally balanced between your heels and toes. Many people like to start with their knees slightly bent to help steady themselves.

- When you find this neutral position, take a couple of breaths to center yourself.

- Once you feel ready, start slowly walking, moving one foot at a time and notice as much of the experience as you can: the feeling of transferring your weight, lifting one foot off the ground, slowly moving it through the air as you balance on the other one, feeling the initial contact with the ground, and equalizing the pressure between the soles of your feet.

- If thoughts or emotions start to occupy your mind, acknowledge them, allow them to drift away, and return your attention to your movements.

- If the distractions persist, you can always take a moment to pause and re-center yourself either in mid-step or with both feet beneath you, before resuming a mindful walk.

- When you reach the end of your walk, take a moment to stand in your initial neutral or balanced standing position. Take two deep breaths and as you exhale the second time, slowly open your eyes.

This is a unique meditation practice because it incorporates physical movement and mindfulness. These are a few examples of the sensations you may notice, and you will begin to experience them in greater details as your awareness expands. Similar to breathing mindfully, walking mindfully can easily be incorporated into your day as a way to quickly reset.

6. LOVING KINDNESS MEDITATION

A meditation on loving kindness or *metta* as it is called in the Buddha's language, Pali, can be a wonderful introduction to cultivating compassion for ourselves and others. This meditation follows a simple progression of sending compassion to various people in your life through visualization coupled with repeating the following mantra of compassion in your mind:

May you know peace.

May you be happy.
May you be loved.
May you be free from suffering.

A mantra is a sound, word, or phrase that is slowly repeated in one's head to help aid concentration. In the context of the loving kindness meditation, you would say this sequence of four sentences in order and then repeat it again in order. It is usually done in the seated position and begins by gently closing your eyes and centering yourself with a few breaths.

There are many ways to start but it typically begins by directing thoughts of loving kindness to yourself first. It is often done by repeating these phrases in your head, replacing "you" with "I" (i.e., "May I know peace," etc.).

- As you repeat this mantra slowly a few times in your head, allow feelings of warmth, care, love, and compassion to fill your body.

- After a few minutes have passed, allow the words to slowly fade as you exhale.

- As you inhale, imagine someone you love standing before you. It can be someone living or passed. When they come into view, slowly repeat the loving kindness mantra to them: May you know peace...

- After a few minutes have passed, allow this person to slowly fade from your mind's eye as you exhale.

- As you inhale, imagine someone you feel somewhat neutral toward standing before you. It can be a coworker with whom you have little interaction or a stranger you passed on the street. When they come into view, slowly repeat the loving kindness mantra to them: May you know peace....

- If it becomes too challenging to send your compassion to this

person (i.e., if you feel your warmth and compassion diminish
rapidly), you can always allow this person to fade away and
return repeating the loving kindness mantra to someone you
love or to yourself.

- After a few minutes have passed, allow this person to slowly fade
from your mind's eye as you exhale.

- As you inhale, imagine someone you feel somewhat negatively
toward standing before you. It can be a person with whom you have
recently had conflict or someone from your more distant past. When
you first begin practicing the metta meditation, I would recommend either skipping this step or imagining someone toward whom
you feel only slightly negative. This is because it can be difficult to
continue to send compassion toward someone for whom you have
strong negative feelings. When they come into view, slowly repeat
the loving kindness mantra to them: May you know peace....

- If it becomes too challenging to send your compassion to this person
(i.e., if you feel your warmth and compassion diminish rapidly), you
can always allow this person to fade away and return to repeating the
loving kindness mantra to someone you love or to yourself.

- After a few minutes have passed, allow this person to slowly fade
from your mind's eye as you exhale.

- As you inhale, imagine all living beings on this planet from small single-
celled organisms to plants, animals, and humans. When all life on this
planet comes into view, slowly repeat the loving kindness mantra to
them: May all living beings know peace....

- After a few minutes have passed, allow the images of all living
beings to slowly fade from your mind's eye as you exhale.

- Return your attention to your breath for a few cycles and notice the steady inhalation and exhalation. Take one more breath, and as you exhale, open your eyes when you're ready.

While I was at a mindfulness conference in 2013, I learned an alternative method to this loving kindness meditation during a break-out session with a doctoral student. Instead of saying these words to ourselves, she had us do the following visualization: *Imagine someone who loves you standing in front of you. It can be someone living or passed away. Once they come into view, you may imagine how they look, what he or she is wearing. As they stand before you, imagine them smiling down on you. Allow their love and compassion to fill you and radiate through you as you hear them say these words: May you know peace...*

What I love about this variation is that the person who I imagine that loves me changes from time to time. When I first tried this exercise, I thought I would visualize my partner, but instead my brother spontaneously appeared in my mind's eye. My partner has often shown up when I have practiced metta since, but it was a wonderful experience of making an unexpected connection while sitting in a conference.

Whichever variant you choose, regularly practicing the loving kindness meditation can be quite beneficial. As you cultivate compassion and awareness, you will lower your stress and improve your happiness during the day, which will ultimately help you fall asleep and stay asleep.

7. PROGRESSIVE MUSCLE RELAXATION (PMR)

This exercise can be done in a seated position, but I suggest lying down if possible. This is not always feasible, especially when in a small office, but lying down allows you to fully tense and fully relax your muscles systematically without having to engage your muscles to sit.

- When you find a comfortable position, allow your eyes to gently close and take a couple of breaths to center yourself.

- When you're ready, clench your right hand into a fist. As you do, notice the tension as it winds its way around your fingers and moves through your hand, past your wrist, and into your forearm.

- After taking a couple of breaths, release the tension from your right arm and notice the cool sensation of relaxation rush down through your arm as you relax your forearm and hand and uncurl your fingers.

- Clench your right hand into a fist again, tighter this time. Notice the warmth and tension surge up through your hand, your wrist, through your forearm, past your elbow, and into your biceps and triceps.

- Notice the tension build as your muscles strain.

- Relax. Notice the cool sensation rush down through your arm as your upper arm, forearm, wrist, and fingers relax.

- From there you can use this basic pattern of flexing certain muscle groups, noticing the tension and warmth this creates, followed by relaxing them and noticing the feeling this creates to relax the rest of your body. You can use the following list as a guide for the progression, but be creative with whatever order works best for you. If there is an area of your body that is too painful to actively clench, feel free to move to another part of your body instead.

- Left arm: do the same as for the right arm.

- Shoulders: squeeze your shoulders together and raise them toward your ears.

- Face: squint your eyes, crinkle your nose, and wrinkle your forehead.

Notice the tension converge on that spot between your eyes.

- Chest: squeeze your chest muscles by drawing your arms together in front of your chest.

- Upper back: apply tension to your upper back by squeezing your shoulder blades together.

- Stomach: clench your stomach muscles.

- Lower back: arch your lower back.

- Legs 1: point your toes away from you. Notice the tension move up through the bottoms of your feet, the backs of your ankles, your calves and into your thighs.

- Legs 2: pull your toes up toward your face this time. Notice the tension move up through the tops of your feet, in front of your ankles, through your shins, and into your thighs.

- After tensing and relaxing the different muscles of your body, take a moment to notice how your body feels as you lie completely relaxed. Take a couple of breaths and slowly open your eyes as you exhale.

PMR is an easy exercise to practice during the evening as you wind down for the night. Even during the day, PMR can easily be done in a few minutes by just picking a few muscles to intentionally tense and relax.

8. VISUALIZATION

Visualization is another great method for relaxation whether it is for sleep, conquering a fear, or to feel calm before a performance.

Depending upon your purpose, there are different ways to go about implementing this exercise. If you are someone trying to reduce your fear of heights, you may start by actually imagining situations that elicit that fear while practicing breathing exercises to relax yourself before trying this in the physical world. This process of graded exposure, or systematic desensitization, is a simple and effective method for dissolving your fear response.

If you are someone using visualization for sleep, imagining a difficult night of sleep often makes you more anxious or frustrated. Instead, visualizing calming scenery is the way to go to help you ease into sleep. The way that I learned this was to have someone decide upon which relaxing environment they would like me to guide them through: a grassy hillside, a path through a forest, a beach, or even through a city. Starting with a few relaxing breaths and progressive muscle relaxation, I would then describe the scenery, touching upon as many senses as possible.

The following is an example of the beginning of a visualization of one of my favorite places to describe: a grassy hillside. It is meant to give you a flavor for how to start and hopefully your imagination will fill in the details.

Imagine you're standing on the side of grassy hillside. It gently slopes down in front of you and levels out into a long flat plain. It rises steeply into mountains at the horizon, pale blue ridges and peaks. The grass around you is knee-high, silvery-green, and tickles your ankles and calves as they rustle in the swirling breeze. A gust of wind blows down from the top of the hill, wrapping around your back, and sending waves through the grass as it weaves away in front of you and across the flatland. Drawing in a deep breath, you smell slightly damp earth as you turn your gaze overhead and close your eyes. You see the reddish-orange glow of the sun through your eyelids and feel it's warmth radiate down your face, shoulders, arms, torso, legs, and into your toes. As you exhale, you drop your gaze to the horizon and slowly open your eyes. A soft silvery haze lifts as your eyes readjust.

9. AUTOGENIC TRAINING

This practice is typically done lying down so you can notice the heaviness in your body. When you find a comfortable position, gently close your eyes and take a couple of deep slow breaths as you settle in.

When you're ready, slowly repeat these phrases in your head:

- My right arm is feeling relaxed and heavy.

- My right arm is feeling heavier and heavier.

- My right arm is completely heavy.

- I feel completely calm.

- After repeating that sequence three times, move to your left arm, both arms, your right leg, left leg, both legs, and finally both arms and both legs.

After practicing that sequence every day for a week, you can then combine it with sending warmth to your arms and legs:

- My right arm is feeling relaxed and warm.

- My right arm is feeling warmer and warmer.

- My right arm is completely warm.

- I feel completely calm.

- After repeating that sequence three times, move to your left arm, both arms, your right leg, left leg, both legs, and finally both arms and both legs.

As you can see, getting through just these first two components of autogenic training can take some time. A few weeks of daily practice is often all that a patient will have time for in CBTi because it is a brief intervention. The full sequence of autogenic training includes the following four sequences, though I have heard from clients that just the first two components (heaviness and warmth) provide a lot of benefit alone.

After practicing the warmth sequence every day for a week, you can then combine it with calming your heart:

- My arms and legs are feeling relaxed and warm.

- My arms and legs are feeling warmer and warmer.

- My arms and legs are completely warm.

- My chest feels warm and relaxed.

- My heartbeat is relaxed and steady.

- I feel completely calm.

After practicing this sequence every day for a week, you can then combine it with relaxing your breathing:

- My arms and legs are feeling relaxed and warm.

- My arms and legs are feeling warmer and warmer.

- My arms and legs are completely warm.

- My heartbeat is relaxed and steady.

- My breathing is calm and steady.

- I feel completely calm.

After practicing this sequence every day for a week, you can then combine it with sending warmth to your stomach:

- My arms and legs are feeling relaxed and warm.

- My arms and legs are feeling warmer and warmer.

- My arms and legs are completely warm.

- My heartbeat is relaxed and steady.

- My breathing is calm and steady.

- My stomach feels soft and warm.

- I feel completely calm.

After practicing this sequence every day for a week, you can then combine it with sending coolness to your forehead:

- My arms and legs are feeling relaxed and warm.

- My arms and legs are feeling warmer and warmer.

- My arms and legs are completely warm.

- My heartbeat is relaxed and steady.

- My breathing is calm and steady.

- My stomach feels soft and warm.

- My forehead feels cool and relaxed.

- I feel completely calm.

Completing the entire sequence of autogenic training takes time and dedication. However, its profoundly positive effects on your body's relaxation response makes it a powerful tool for helping you feel relaxed enough to get fall asleep."

RECOMMENDED RESOURCES

BOOKS

Jon Kabat-Zinn. *Full Catastrophe Living: Using the Wisdom of Your Body and Mind to Face Stress, Pain, and Illness*. New York: Dell, 1991.

Jon Kabat-Zinn. *Wherever You Go, There You Are*. New York: Hyperion Books, 1994.

Marie Kondo. *The Life-Changing Magic of Tidying Up: The Japanese Art of Decluttering and Organizing*. Ten Speed Press, 2014.

Meir H. Kryger, Thomas Roth, and William C. Dement. *Principles & Practice of Sleep Medicine, 5th Edition*. St. Louis, MO: Saunders, 2010.

Michael Pollan. *In Defense of Food: An Eater's Manifesto*. New York: Penguin Press, 2008.

Tony Schwartz. *The Way We're Working Isn't Working*. New York: Free Press, 2010.

Shauna L. Shapiro and Linda E. Carlson, *The Art and Science of Mindfulness: Integrating Mindfulness into Psychology and the Helping Professions*. Washington, DC: American Psychological Association, 2009.

Justin Sonnenburg and Erica Sonnenburg. *The Good Gut: Taking Control of Your Weight, Your Mood, and Your Longer-term Health*. New York: Penguin, 2015.

WEBSITES

History of Sleep: Harvard Medical School:
http://healthysleep.med.harvard.edu/healthy/matters/history

How Long to Nap: http://www.wsj.com/news/interactive/SLEEP0902

Free Mindfulness-based stress reduction (MBSR) resources and information:

- Palouse Mindfulness: http://palousemindfulness.com/index.html

- UCLA Mindful Awareness Research Center: http://marc.ucla.edu/body.
  cfm?id=22

- UCSD Center for Mindfulness: https://health.ucsd.edu/specialties/
  mindfulness/programs/mbsr/Pages/audio.aspx

- BYU Counseling and Psychological Services: https://caps.byu.edu/audio-files

Diagnosis and Treatment of Sleep Disorders:

- The Stanford Center: http://sleep.stanford.edu

APPS

Insight Timer
Headspace
MindShift
Mindfulness Coach
ACT Coach
CBTi Coach
Jetlagrooster

NOTES

1   Brené Brown, *The Gift of Imperfection: Let Go of Who You Think You're Supposed to Be and Embrace Who You Are* (Center City, MN: Hazelden, 2010).

2   Charles Morin & Colin Espie, as cited in *The Oxford Handbook of Sleep and Sleep Disorders* (Oxford Press, New York, NY: Oxford Handbooks Online, 2016).

3   Bryce A Mander, Shawn M Marks, Jacob W Vogel, Vikram Rao, Brandon Lu, Jared M Saletin, Sonia Ancoli-Israel, William J Jagust & Matthew P Walker (2015). Beta-amyloid disrupts human NREM slow waves and related hippocampus-dependent memory consolidation. *Nature Neuroscience*, 18(7), 1051-1057. doi:10.1038/nn.4035

4   Bio, accessed on 09/11/16, http://www.biography.com/people/aristotle-9188415.

5   Thich Nhat Hanh, *Plum Village Chanting and Recitation Book*. (Berkeley, CA: Parallax Press, 2000).

6   The Golden Circle, accessed on 09/11/16, http://image.slidesharecdn.com/simon-sinek-thegoldencircle-140721045441-phpapp02/95/simon-sinek-the-golden-circle-start-with-the-why-6-638.jpg?cb=1405918613.

7   Plum Village, accessed on 09/11/16, http://plumvillage.org/retreats/info/ireland-wake-up-retreat-2016/.

8   "A Letter From Our Founder," The Center for Compassion and Altruism Research and Education, accessed on 09/11/16, http://ccare.stanford.edu/education/about-compassion-cultivation-training-cct/a-letter-from-our-founder/.

BIBLIOGRAPHY

"A Letter From Our Founder," The Center for Compassion and Altruism Research and Education, accessed 05/30/2016, http://ccare.stanford.edu/education/about-compassion-cultivation-training-cct/a-letter-from-our-founder/.

Åkerstedt, Torbjörn, and Folkard, Simon. "The Three-Process Model of Alertness and Its Extension to Performance, Sleep Latency, and Sleep Length." *Chronobiology International*, 14 (1997): 115–123.

Berridge, Kent C., and Robinson, Terry E. "What Is the Role of Dopamine in Reward: Hedonic Impact, Reward Learning, or Incentive Salience?" *Brain Research Reviews*, 28 (1998). 309–369.

Borbély, Alexander A. "A Two Process Model of Sleep Regulation." *Human Neurobiology*, 1 (1982): 195–204.

Burns, David D. *Feeling Good: The New Mood Therapy*. New York: HarperCollins, 1999.

Cappuccio, Francesco P., Taggart, Frances M., Kandala, Ngianga-Bakwin, Currie, Andrew, Peile, Ed, Stranges, Saverio, and Miller, Michelle A. "Meta-Analysis of Short Sleep Duration and Obesity in Children and Adults," *Sleep*, 31 (2008): 619–626.

Carney, Collen E., Buysse, Daniel J., Ancoli-Israel, Sonia, Edinger, Jack D., Krystal, Andrew D., Lichstein, Kenneth L., and Morin, Charles N. "The Consensus Sleep Diary: Standardizing Prospective Sleep Self-Monitoring," *Sleep*, 35 (2012): 287–302.

De Koninck, Joseph-Marie, Christ, Günter, Hébert, Guy, and Rinfret, Natalie "Language Learning Efficiency, Dreams and REM Sleep," *Psychiatric Journal of the University of Ottawa*, 15 (1990): 91–92.

De Koninck, Joseph-Marie, Lorrain, Dominique, Christ, Günter, Proulx, Geneviève, and Coulombe, Daniel "Intensive Language Learning and Increases in Rapid Eye Movement Sleep: Evidence of a Performance Factor," *International Journal of Psychophysiology*, 8 (1989): 43–47.

Durgan, David, Ganesh, Bhanu, Cope, Julia, Ajami, Nadim, Phillips, Sharon, Petrosino, Joseph, Hollister, Emily, and Bryna, Robert, "Role of the Gut Microbiome in Obstructive Sleep Apnea-Induced Hypertension," *Hypertension*, 67 (2016): 469–474.

Gais, Steffen, Mölle, Matthias, Helms, Kay, and Born, Jan, "Learning-Dependent Increases in Sleep Spindle Density," *The Journal of Neuroscience*, 22 (2002): 6830–6834.

Gau, Susan Shur-Fen, Shang, Chi-Yung, Merikangas, Kathleen Ries, Chiu, Yen-Nan., Soong, Wiely T., and Cheng, Andrew T. A. "Association Between Morningness-Eveningness and Behavioral/Emotional Problems Among Adolescents," *Journal of Biological Rhythms*, 22 (2007): 268–274.

Goldstein-Piekarski, Andrea N., Greer, Stephanie M., Saletin, Jared M., and Walker, Matthew P. "Sleep Deprivation Impairs the Human Central and Peripheral Nervous System Discrimination of Social Threat," *The Journal of Neuroscience*, 35 (2015): 10135–10145.

Gollwitzer, Peter M. "Implementation Intentions: Strong Effects of Simple Plans," *American Psychologist*, 54 (1999): 493–503.

Herwig, Uwe, Kaffenberger, Karen, Jäncke, Lutz, and Brühl, Annette B., "Self-Related Awareness and Emotion Regulation," *NeuroImage*, 50 (2010): 734–741.

Jazaieri, Hooria, McGonigal, Kelly, Jinpa, Thupten, Doty, James R., Gross, James J., and Golden, Philippe R. "A Randomized Controlled Trial of Compassion Cultivation Training: Effects on Mindfulness, Affect, and Emotion Regulation," *Motivation and Emotion*, 38 (2014): 23–35.

Kabat-Zinn, Jon. *Wherever You Go, There You Are*. New York: Hyperion Books, 1994.

Lally, Phillippa, van Jaarsveld, Cornelia H. M., Potts, Henry W. W., and Wardle, Jane. "How are Habits Formed: Modelling Habit Formation in the Real World," *European Journal of Social Psychology*, 6 (2010): 998–1009.

Mah, Cheri D., Mah, Kenneth E., Kezirian, Eric J., and Dement, William C. "The Effects of Sleep Extension on the Athletic Performance of Collegiate Basketball Players," *Sleep*, 34 (2011): 943–950.

Mander, Bryce A., Marks, Shawn M., Vogel, Jacob W., Rao, Vikram, Lu, Brandon, Saletin, Jared M., Ancoli-Israel, Sonia, Jagust, William J., and Walker, Matthew P. "Ð-Amyloid Disrupts Human NREM Slow Waves and Related Hippocampus-Dependent Memory Consolidation," *Nature Neuroscience*, 18 (2015): 1051–1057.

Mauvieux, Benoît, Gouthière, Laurent, Sesboüe, Bruno, and Davenne, Damien "A Study Comparing Circadian Rhythm and Sleep Quality of Athletes and Sedentary Subjects Engaged in Night Work," *Canadian Journal of Applied Physiology*, 28 (2003): 831–887. [Article in French].

Mullington, Janet M., Simpson, Norah S., Meier-Ewert, Hans K., and Haack, Monika "Sleep Loss and Inflammation," *Best Practice & Research: Clinical Endocrinology & Metabolism*, 24 (2010): 775–784.

Neckelmann, Dag, Mykletun, Amstein, and Dahl, Alv A. "Chronic Insomnia as a Risk Factor for Developing Anxiety and Depression," *Sleep*, 30 (2007): 873–880.

Nishida, Masaki, Pearsall, Jori, Buckner, Randy L., and Walker, Matthew P. "REM Sleep, Prefrontal Theta, and the Consolidation of Human Emotional Memory," *Cerebral Cortex*, 19 (2009): 1158–1166.

Passos, Giselle S., Poyares, Dalva, Santana, Marcos G., D'Aurea, Carolina V.R., Youngstedt, Shawn D., Tufik, Sergio, and de Mello, Marco T. "Effects of Moderate Aerobic Exercise Training on Chronic Primary Insomnia," *Sleep Medicine*, 12 (2011): 1018–1027.

Rechtschaffen, Allen. "The Control of Sleep." In *Human Behavior and Its Control*, edited by William A. Hunt, 75–92. Cambridge: Schenkman, 1971.

Reid, Kathryn J., Baron, Kelly B., Lu, Brandon, Naylor, Eric, Wolfe, Lisa, and Zee, Phyliis C. "Aerobic Exercise Improves Self-Reported Sleep and Quality of Life in Older Adults with Insomnia," *Sleep Medicine*, 11 (2010): 934–940.

Sakami, Shotaro, Ishikawa, Toshio, Kawakami, Norito, Haratani, Takashi, Fukui, Akira, Kobayashi, Fumio, Fujita, Osamu, Araki, Shunichi, and Kawamura, Noriyuki "Coemergence of Insomnia and a Shift in the Th1/Th2 balance Toward Th2 Dominance," *Neuroimmunomodulation*, (2001-2003): 337–343.

Shakhar, Keren, Valdimarsdottir, Heiddis B., Guevarra, Josephine S., and Bovbjerg, Dana H. "Sleep, Fatigue, and NK Cell Activity in Healthy Volunteers: Significant Relationships Revealed by Within Subject Analyses," *Brain, Behavior, and Immunity*, (2007): 180–184.

Shapiro, Shauna L and Carlson, Linda E. *The Art and Science of Mindfulness: Integrating Mindfulness into Psychology and the Helping Professions.* Washington, DC: American Psychological Association, 2009.

Sinek, Simon. *Start with Why: How Great Leaders Inspire Everyone to Take Action.* New York: Portfolio, 2011.

Sonnenburg, Justin, and Sonnenburg, Erica. *The Good Gut: Taking Control of Your Weight, Your Mood, and Your Longer-term Health.* New York: Penguin, 2015.

Spielman, Arthur J., and Glovinsky, Paul B. "The Varied Nature of Insomnia." In *Case Studies in Insomnia*, edited by Peter J. Hauri, 1–15. New York: Plenum Press, 1991.

St-Onge, Marie-Pierre, Roberts, Amy, Shechter, Ari, and Choudhury, Arindam R. "Fiber and Saturated Fat Are Associated with Sleep Arousals and Slow Wave Sleep," *Journal of Clinical Sleep Medicine,* 12 (2016): 19–24.

Teasdale, John D. "Metacognition, Mindfulness and the Modification of Mood Disorders," *Clinical Psychology and Psychotherapy,* 6 (1999):146–155.

Walker, Matthew, Brakefield, Tiffany, Morgan, Alexandra, Hobson, J. Allen, and Stickgold, Robert "Practice with Sleep Makes Perfect: Sleep-Dependent Motor Skill Learning," *Neuron,* 35 (2002): 205–211.

Wright, Caroline E., Erblich, Joel, Valdimarsdottir, Heiddis B., and Bovbjerg, Dana H. "Poor Sleep the Night Before an Experimental Stressor Predicts Reduced NK Cell Mobilization and Slowed Recovery in Healthy Women," *Brain, Behavior, and Immunity,* 21 (2007): 358–363.

Yang, Pei-Yu, Ho, Ka-Hou, Chen, His-Chung, and Chien, Meng-Yueh "Exercise Training Improves Sleep Quality in Middle-Aged and Older Adults with Sleep Problems: A Systematic Review," *Journal of Physiotherapy,* 58 (2012): 157–163.

Youngstedt, Shawn D. "Effects of Exercise on Sleep," *Clinics in Sports Medicine,* 24 (2005): 355–365.

Youssef, Nagy A., Ege, Margaret, Angly, Sohair S., Strauss, Jennifer L., and Marx, Christine E. "Is Obstructive Sleep Apnea Associated with ADHD?" *Annals of Clinical Psychiatry,* 23 (2011): 213–224.

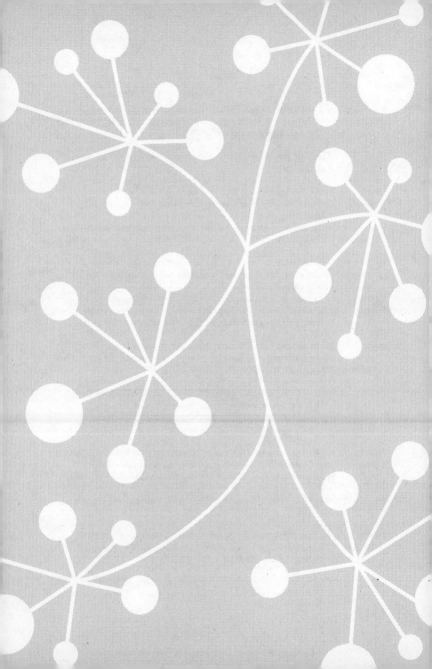

ACKNOWLEDGMENTS

There are so many people who I would like to thank for the inspiration and opportunity to write this book. To all my sleep mentors: Dr. Ilona Vail, Dr. Paula Andrasi, Dr. Allison Harvey, Nancee Zannone, Dr. Fiona Barwick, and Dr. Allison Siebern. Each one of you helped spark and nurture my passion for sleep health. To the team at Parallax Press, particularly Jason Kim: your belief in and enthusiasm for my approach to healthy sleep practices made this book a reality. To Al and Sari: your mindful editing was crucial in the eleventh hour. Last and certainly not least to my partner, Emily—you blazed the trail toward improving our sleep, provided the focused encouragement that allowed me to pursue this field of sleep health that I love, and offered your partnership in this book. Thank you all. You have my deepest gratitude.

RELATED TITLES

Awakening Joy, James Baraz and Shoshana Alexander

Deep Relaxation, Sister Chan Khong

Happiness, Thich Nhat Hanh

How to Sit, Thich Nhat Hanh

Making Space, Thich Nhat Hanh

The Mindful Athlete, George Mumford

Mindfulness as Medicine, Sister Dang Nghiem

Nothing to It, Brother Phap Hai

Ten Breaths to Happiness, Glen Schneider

ABOUT THE AUTHORS

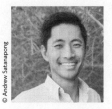

Daniel Jin Blum, PhD is a licensed clinical psychologist who specializes in sleep health. He is a former sleep coach at University of California Berkeley and Behavioral Sleep Medicine Fellow at The Stanford Sleep Center. Dr. Blum lives in San Francisco where he is a staff psychologist at Square and maintains a private practice.

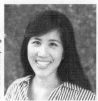

Emily Tsiang is a Life Design Fellow at Stanford and Senior Facilitator with The Energy Project. She catalyzes people and organizations by harnessing the science of high performance.